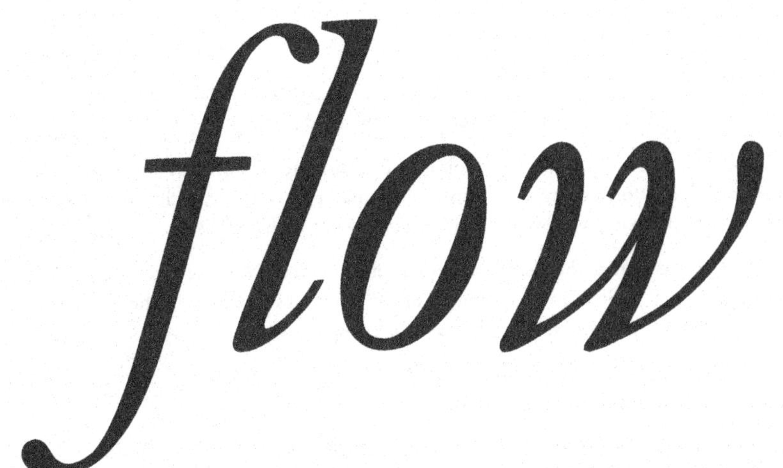

flow

GROWING A SPIRITUAL Yoga Practice in Church

Susan W. Springer
with Sirena Dudgeon

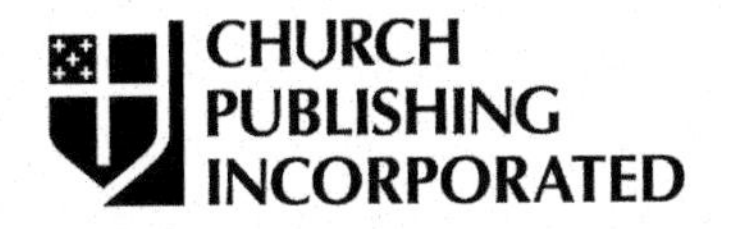
CHURCH PUBLISHING INCORPORATED

Church Publishing
19 East 34th Street
New York, NY 10016

Cover design by Dylan Marcus McConnell, Tiny Little Hammers
Typeset by Rose Design

Library of Congress Cataloging-in-Publication Data

Names: Springer, Susan W., author.
Title: Flow : growing a spiritual yoga practice in church / Susan W. Springer with Sirena Dudgeon.
Description: New York, NY : Church Publishing, [2022] | Includes bibliographical references.
Identifiers: LCCN 2021048207 (print) | LCCN 2021048208 (ebook) | ISBN 9781640653535 (paperback) | ISBN 9781640653542 (ebook)
Subjects: LCSH: Christianity and yoga.
Classification: LCC BR128.Y63 S67 2022 (print) | LCC BR128.Y63 (ebook) | DDC 294.5/436--dc23/eng/20211115
LC record available at https://lccn.loc.gov/2021048207
LC ebook record available at https://lccn.loc.gov/2021048208

CONTENTS

INTRODUCTION

Skeptical but Desperate

Name a sport, and I've probably pursued it: from back-country skiing to paragliding, from cycling to golf, from trail running to kayaking. As an adult I've lived in places like Maine, Alaska, and the Rocky Mountains that are conducive to outdoor sports. I was working as an Episcopal priest in Boulder, Colorado, and playing outdoors as much as I could when a couple of car accidents changed that. As I convalesced, my body hurt trying to do all that it had done before, and I watched myself grow more sedentary. One day, in desperation, I tried yoga.

To say I had an unmerited bias against yoga would be an understatement. Boulder is something of a yoga mecca, where studios abound, and people get dreamy-eyed talking about their favorite teacher. Yoga festivals, schools, and clothing retailers mark every block of the downtown. Yoga talk and Buddhist terms thread themselves through casual conversation. Earnest and wispy young practitioners bicycle about, with dreadlocks flying and tanned, tattooed arms clutching rolled-up mats. As a dread-less, tatt-less older person, I had always determined that yoga was not for me. As one who felt her flexibility, agility, and balance were pretty darn good for a late-middle-aged woman, I had always assumed yoga would not be much of a challenge. As someone more drawn to speed than silence, I had always thought that yoga would be b-o-r-i-n-g. And as a second-generation cradle Episcopalian, I didn't think my theology and spiritual practice needed any accessorizing.

On all counts, I could not have been more wrong.

A fellow yoga-virgin friend and I went to our first class together. It was a community drop-in class open to all levels of practitioners, held after hours in a bike shop. For me, that was a promising sign. Sirena, the teacher, greeted us warmly. I sized her up. Namaste T-shirt? Check. Tattoo? Check. But that was as far as I could take the stereotype. Cascades of blond ringlets framed a blue-eyed cherub face, and the body before me was not wispy—it was a real, lived-in, birthed-two-children body. I was intrigued. Sirena offered the kind of welcoming persona we church leaders seek to offer: genuine, calm, warm, approachable. Ten minutes into my first class, it occurred to me that I had—ahem—*substantially* overrated my flexibility, agility, and balance. Still, embracing the challenge, I made it through and resolved to come again. And I did. That was five years ago, and I am still practicing.

This book is, in part, the story of how—as my body was learning to fold itself into impossible positions (asanas)—my heart was learning to *unfold* itself to see the congruence of yogic philosophy with Christianity. From there, I became inspired to engage Sirena and with her offer yoga in the church I was serving, inviting people in to place their yoga mats on the 117-year-old floor in the lofty and beautiful main worship space of St. John's Episcopal Church in downtown Boulder. Sirena led the flows (the series of asanas), and we took turns exploring a given topic from the perspectives of progressive, mystical Christian theology and the yoga sutras and other yogic philosophies. We want to offer you a template for how you can begin a yoga ministry in your church and why you should seriously consider it. This is not a journey I anticipated. Few good and holy journeys are.

The White-Leafed Turning Point

Every significant journey has a turning point, a place where something (often momentous) happens and the traveler confronts a choice about how to proceed. For me that point was quite specific: Monday night bike shop yoga on July 23, 2018. I realize that Methodists more often than Episcopalians can point to the day and time of their heart-strangely-warmed conversion. What can I say? It happened, evidence that the Holy Spirit is not bound by the denominational particularities we observe.

It was the end of class, and we were easing into *savasana*, the final resting pose that typically ends a session of yoga. Sirena cued up a gorgeous chant in Sanskrit performed by a female vocalist as she led us into a short, guided meditation. I remember wishing she would stop talking so I could lose myself in the music, and I remember she said something about getting out of our own way. Without much conscious effort, I proceeded to do just that, and what happened next was extraordinary.

I imagined myself—the ego me—climbing out of my heart-space and crouching at the right side of my supine body to watch. That conscious imagining took just a moment before I became not the thinker or the doer but simply the observer. In astonishment I watched my chest open, the layers of skin and flesh and bone parting bloodlessly, as a white vine at least six inches in diameter began to rise. It was made of a stuff I'd never seen before, closed-cell spongey like the stem of a forest mushroom but shimmering silver and wet. Fascinated—and, frankly, slightly freaked out—I watched it rise toward the ceiling of the bike shop, lazily winding its way upward through space. I'm not sure how it penetrated the roof or the trees or the power lines, because in the next image the vine and I were spiraling up through what meteorologists would call the *troposphere*—the highest level of altitude to which passenger jets climb and fly. We ascended through layers of clouds stained apricot and purple by the setting sun. It was beautiful and peaceful.

I looked up to see a canopy of white, heart-shaped leaves extend from the vine in all directions. It was the kind of sudden beauty that makes you gasp. I remember a moment of worry that this marked the end of the vision, but it did not. The vine continued its upward climb, and it was then I began to understand where I was going and into whose presence I was entering. Suddenly, I was washed and held in a golden-colored familial love so deep and profound it was pure ecstasy. All the human and canine loves I've ever experienced, added up and multiplied a hundredfold, could not begin to approach its power. The God I encountered was not Hindu or Christian or the property of any religion. I began to weep at the joy and the relief of it. A second canopy of leaves shot out from the vine, and then Sirena's voice called us back to the awareness of our bodies on our mats. Moments later, as I made my way to a sitting position for our final prayer *mudra* and gentle bow, my face and throat were wet and my eyes continued to cascade tears.

I love my church and cannot imagine being anything but an Episcopalian; however, little in my Episcopal worship or spiritual experience has ever, ever come close to touching the unmitigated communion with the divine I experienced that day. What did it all mean? I'm still not sure, but I do know stuff like that doesn't typically happen to me on a Monday night.

A Journey of Discovery

In the months that followed I began to dig deeper into the yoga sutras and ancient Indian religious texts like the Upanishads and the Bhagavad Gita. Every time an ancient saying called to mind the words or the teachings of Jesus or Paul, I scribbled a note to myself in the margins. The pages of my books became littered with notes on the parallels between Christian theology and yogic philosophy. As Sirena and I offered class after class on topics like surrender, anxiety, and community, I realized I was only scratching the surface of all that the two traditions hold in common.

I am far from the first Christian to experience the divine on a yoga mat or to ponder the intersection of yoga and Christianity. Both yoga and Christianity seek to experience communion with the divine and a deepening relationship or identity with the divine. Numerous forms of "Christian yoga," as well as Christian yoga teacher training schools, have arisen. For me these run the risk of melding two important traditions that do not ask to become one—two rivers that each flow with great integrity on their own, even though they eventually empty into the same sea. This book doesn't seek to Christianize yoga or yoga-ize Christianity. Rather, it endeavors to notice and appreciate the points of connection between the Yoga Sutras of Patanjali and other ancient Indian religious texts with progressive, mystical Christian theology.

I define progressive, mystical Christian theology[1] as that which sees the divine in all things, even (taking a page from quantum physics) in all matter, both animate and inanimate; that does not discount nor minimize the pervasiveness or seriousness of sin and evil but that nonetheless regards human beings as inherently good as opposed to inherently sinful; that humbly acknowledges that Christianity does not have an exclusive claim on the divine nor the only way to experience communion with the divine; that honors tradition while embracing change—even when discomforting; that finds love to be at the heart of God and love to be the divine nature of God; that values contemplative practice as a way of experiencing union with the divine; and that upholds the individual believer's capacity for divine encounter, unmediated by an ordained cleric or the institution she serves.

I propose that the common teachings of yoga and Christianity can build a framework within which the church can reach out to those who do not know us and who perhaps have never heard of the progressive, mystical stream within Christianity. If yoga in the church is to be a form of evangelism (a gentle doorway into the church or the gentle planting of a seed), then church leaders need to acknowledge they have much repair work to do before they can expect yoga practitioners to become church members. The religious experience of many people is riddled with wounds; their paths are potholed with harmful experiences of institutional religion. Yoga in the church is a way to say quietly, "The judgmental, hypocritical, exclusivist church of your

---

1. My principal guides in this theology include Richard Rohr and his work on the Cosmic or Universal Christ, John Philip Newell and his work on Celtic Christian spirituality, and Pierre Teilhard de Chardin and his work on both love and the collective journey of humanity (and creation) toward the Omega Point. Christian scriptures that appear to particularly lend themselves to this conversation include the Gospel of John and the Epistles of Paul, although passages from Hebrew scripture have bearing as well.

upbringing is not who we aspire to be, and in fact to the extent we have been that church, we repent."

There are many places where Hinduism (the tradition to which yoga was first bound) and Christianity do *not* align, and this book does not try to make them do so. Instead, it seeks to identify and explore those places where yogic philosophy and Christian theology are saying the same things about God and the human experience.

I am motivated in part by a talk I once heard Richard Rohr give to the Episcopal clergy of Colorado at our annual retreat. Rohr declared that clergy do a great job of telling people what to believe and a terrible job of teaching people how to live. I've not forgotten his harsh—but true—observation. For me the yoga sutras offer a springboard into the teachings of Jesus—teachings that give his followers a way to live. The church (if it is to survive) can no longer be an institution where one is either in or out according to the measure of one's right belief but instead must be reimagined as a school for learning how to love: how to love self, creation, others, and God.[2]

In 2019, the Louisville Institute awarded me a Pastoral Study Project grant to explore and write about the intersections of yogic philosophy with Christian scripture and theology. As part of that grant, I completed my 200-hour yoga teacher training at the Kripalu Center for Yoga and Health in Massachusetts. Through all this, Sirena has been my partner in discovery, albeit from a very different background and perspective, and she has cheered me forward. I feel honored to have shared these miles with her.

Recovering Catholic Yoga Teacher Meets Priest: An Introduction by Sirena Dudgeon

Having been raised Roman Catholic in a small northern Indiana town, I found a deep love and respect for spiritual ritual as a way to connect with God. Starting from a young age, I found solace and comfort praying the rosary, singing in the church choir, and helping my grandfather as an usher during Mass. I participated in church school every Wednesday evening and helped my mom teach the preschooler's Sunday school class. As my interest in spirituality grew, I sought to deepen my knowledge of religious and spiritual philosophy by reading books and participating in meetings for other religious and spiritual

2. For more on church as a school for learning how to love: Brian McLaren, *The Great Spiritual Migration* (New York: Convergent Books, 2016), 50–66.

communities. In college at the University of Northern Colorado, I attended my first yoga class to help balance the stresses of studying and working. This experience provided me a different kind of connection to God—through my body. I had played many sports in my younger years but had never experienced anything like yoga. I was deeply drawn to understanding how and why yoga asana and pranayama could elevate, uplift, and connect my mind, body, and spirit.

As a long-time student of asana and meditation practice, I yearned for more in my yoga journey. I completed my 200-hour Yoga Alliance Certified Teacher Training at Full Circle Yoga in Longmont, Colorado, in 2016. This immediately opened my path to everything the eight limbs of yoga had to offer: mantra, sutras, anatomy, spirituality, ritual, and yogic scripture. Soon after graduation, I started my first teaching job on Monday nights at a community bike shop. This class was held on a bicycle grease–spattered floor, surrounded by high-end bicycles, tires, and helmets, and was intended to present yoga as nothing more than an exercise regimen good for cyclists. I stayed true to the ancient roots of the yogic philosophy and wove the spiritual aspect of it into my flows. I soon established a following of regular students who came weekly to connect, laugh, breathe, and move their bodies. It was the spiritual community I knew I had been longing for but hadn't experienced since childhood. Making lasting friendships and deep connections, this bike shop "Zen Den" became my church.

I met Rev. Susan in this Monday night class. She has curly hair just like mine, laughter that lifts all spirits, a positive attitude, and is a gentle nurturer. She brought her friends to class to try yoga. I love meeting new people and especially those new to yoga; I want to make it accessible, approachable, and relatable. I knew there was something very special about Susan when I met her. Her love for God was especially apparent, and even though I was quite hesitant to share my own feelings about God in class, I gently introduced the topic and was able to open up. It was then that I found out Susan was a priest. As a former Catholic, I'd been taught to regard priests as channels to God. I'd also been taught to fear them, and we were rarely allowed to talk to them. But here was Susan—a priest and a woman! I was excited to learn the Episcopal Church permits women to be priests, and I felt a hope and healing coming into my heart.

Often, at the end of class, Susan would connect my theme to a Christian text or teaching. Susan's voice shattered the glass ceiling of my childhood experiences and allowed me room to explore and feel safe and supported in my curiosity. In the library one winter day, I found *Sophia Rising* by Monette Chilson. This book explains how yoga practitioners from any faith can use yoga and its inner wisdom (in Greek, *Sophia*) to create a sacred space inside themselves. It also argues that yogic philosophy and Christian theology are not incompatible. I shared the book with Susan, and we came up with a plan for Yoga in the Church, a series of workshops in which we would offer our own explorations of the meeting places between yogic philosophy and Christian theology. We hoped to share these workshops with Susan's church community as well as people from the wider community. When they see our deep respect for both yoga and Christianity, many of our students have experienced profound healing.

As the Bhagavad Gita states, "Yoga is a journey of the Self, Through the Self, To the Self." I am deeply moved to see Susan grow and blossom in her yoga journey, having completed her 200-hour yoga teacher training. I am honored to be on this path together, sharing our love of God, spiritual teachings, and offering this beautiful moving practice in community. Forever a guiding light in my heart, Susan is a beacon of hope. It is our hope that this book will offer encouragement to all yoga practitioners as we discover together that there is one truth with many paths, guided by love and compassion.

A Pandemic Poses a Challenge

The irony of writing a book on yoga as a creative way to invite people into church worship spaces at the *very moment* in history when the Covid-19 pandemic has sent most of us fleeing from such gathering spaces is not lost on me. The word *pivot* seems to be popping up everywhere to describe how people and institutions are adapting to an unwanted new reality. With Yoga in the Church, we pivoted at the start of the pandemic to move our workshops online. Sirena and I teach on Zoom from our respective homes and not from the church, because it makes no sense to us to invite people to a space we can access but they cannot. We acknowledge, however, that other churches offering online-only workshops may wish to livestream from their worship spaces to make the theological statement that doing yoga in a worship space is a perfectly acceptable way of seeking union with God.

Regardless of the location you choose, you can still offer compelling teaching that examines the points of connection between yogic philosophy and Christian theology. You can still wrap your workshops in beautiful sacred music and can create a reverent space in your home. And you can still extend an invitation to participants to visit the online worship services, classes, fellowship groups, and social justice initiatives your church offers. We say more about this in chapter 4.

Writing this book now also serves as a witness to the resilience of the Christian spirit. We believe this pandemic does not represent the end of church life as we have known it but rather a beginning. Sustained by a belief in the unending cycle of resurrection that marks the nature of individuals, institutions, and creation itself, we look ahead to rebirth and transformation even as we walk through a season of decline. To mix in some scripture, even though we walk through a valley shadowed by death, we acknowledge that everything old has passed away, and we see that everything is becoming new.[3] It is this faith in the resurrection cycle that sustains us and gives us the confidence to offer you our work.

How to Use This Book

Chapters 1 and 2 make a case for the introduction of yoga into a church's ministry life. Chapter 3 digs in to yogic and Christian texts and presents parallel teachings to whet your appetite. Chapter 4 offers instructions on how to prepare a congregation for this new ministry and practical tips on how to build it. Chapter 5 provides customizable guidelines for a year's worth of monthly Yoga in the Church workshops. Chapter 6 shares some stories from the field—interviews with others from Episcopal churches around the country who have already built yoga into their church ministries. We end by reflecting on what else, beyond yoga, God might be doing in the world outside the church doors and by asking how we might join in that work with God.

3. Ps. 23:4; 2 Cor. 5:17.

1

CROSSING TRAJECTORIES

The word *yoga*, as most of you doubtless know, is the same as our word *yoke*. Y-O-K-E. And the Latin word *iungere*, to join. Join, junction, yoke, union, all these words are basically from the same root. And so likewise when Jesus said my yoke is easy, he was saying really my yoga is easy. And the word therefore basically denotes the state that would be the opposite of what our psychologists call alienation: the view of separateness, the feeling of separateness, the feeling of being cut off from being.

–Alan Watts, former Episcopal priest, "Intellectual Yoga"[1]

The End of One Journey Is the Beginning of the Next

The Episcopal Church has been bleeding members in the last fifty years. In that same period, the rise of yoga practitioners in the United States has been remarkable.

In 1958, when I was born into a loyal Episcopalian household, my denomination boasted nearly 3.5 million members. By the time I was ten, I sang enthusiastically in the children's choir every Sunday, but the Church had lost around 100,000 people. And no—those two facts are not related! By the time I was twenty, we had lost seven times that many members. By the time I was thirty, our losses exceeded one million people; by age forty, 1.8 million. In 2008, when I turned fifty, we had happily gained back 300,000 folks, only to lose them—plus an additional 80,000—by 2018.[2] Over the course of my lifetime, the Episcopal Church has shrunk by almost half. My spiritual identity and home are in the Episcopal Church. I truly can't imagine being anything but an Episcopalian and therefore find our dwindling numbers distressing.

1. Alan Watts, "Intellectual Yoga," Alan Watts Organization, April 16, 2019, *https://www.alanwatts.org/1-2-12-intellectual-yoga/*.

2. These figures can be found by reading the *Journals of General Convention* for the years specified: "Journals of General Convention," The Archives of the Episcopal Church, accessed October 14, 2021, *https://www.episcopalarchives.org/governance-documents/journals-of-gc*.

In the glory days of mainline Protestantism, it seemed everyone went to church on Sundays, and families gathered afterward for midday dinner. In New England, where I was raised, the rhythm of it was as dependable as the rise and fall of the tide. The world is different now. Religion in America has all but died to its old way of being—and yet it's needed now as much as it ever has been.

We can cling to a nostalgic view of the past and strive to re-create it, or we can acknowledge in faith that God is urging us to explore new ways of being the body of Christ. I believe that God is dynamic and not static, and, as one earthly manifestation of God, faith communities are called to be likewise—to be aware, responsive, agile, and connected to the life that is unfolding in the towns and cities in which they reside. I believe that the very same Holy Spirit who breathed life into the void at the dawn of creation, who whispered in the ears of prophets, and who was exhaled from the lips of Jesus onto his disciples, is alive and well in the world today and continually dances before the faces of the faithful and faithless alike, to draw our attention to where God would have it land.

If one believes in the presence and power of this Spirit, then it isn't a big leap to assert that parishes in decline are not necessarily dying but rather are in the process of being transformed. Because the Spirit is in the business of bestowing aliveness, transformation may include some dying, but it always also includes some resurrection. Nationwide, Episcopal congregations are aging and declining, and yet that downward trajectory is at this moment crossing with another upward-arcing trajectory: the emergence of a new manifestation of Christianity.[3] If we want to be involved with this new life the Spirit is bringing forth, we must make a conscious choice to be humble and curious instead of woeful and complacent.

What exactly is this "new manifestation of Christianity?" One possible answer is that it's a faith that may still be denominationally loyal but tends to be less denominationally bound, less convinced that its doctrines are the only and best right answer for all situations, and more open to considering the gifts that other faith traditions can offer. This new manifestation of Christianity acknowledges that there is no "perfect" religion and that Christians can sometimes learn a great deal about how to live as Christians by studying people of *other faiths*. It's good for us to be challenged to look beneath the surface of our Christian traditions, creeds, sacraments, and liturgies to find the values that connect us with practitioners of religions unlike our own. Karen Armstrong

3. Insights shared with the author from The Rt. Rev. Rob O'Neill, Tenth Bishop of the Episcopal Diocese of Colorado, personal conversation, December 2017.

did this kind of deep dive in her groundbreaking and award-winning Charter for Compassion.[4]

In the charter and the book that gave rise to it, *Twelve Steps to a Compassionate Life*,[5] Armstrong points out that common moral emphases, as well as a yearning for union with the divine—with divine wisdom—are found in Judaism, Christianity, Islam, Hinduism, and Buddhism. I met and spent the day with Karen Armstrong in 2005, several years before her work on the charter. She was in Ketchum, Idaho, to share a stage with the Dalai Lama, and it was the first exposure to interfaith dialogue I'd had.

I had been assigned to take Ms. Armstrong to lunch and drive her afterward wherever she wished to go. I had been warned that she would probably not want to visit and chat, preferring to retire to her room to rest and prepare. I was surprised and delighted when she proved this advice wrong, lingering over lunch for hours. After the better part of a day, we said our farewells. Our conversation had been exhilarating, but toward the end I had run through every original thought in my brain. I had scraped the bottom of my barrel and had nothing intelligent left to say. As for Armstrong, I suspect she was just getting warmed up. The encounter taught me how sheltered I'd been and how much I had to learn about my brothers and sisters in different faith traditions. My Episcopal upbringing had been snug—even smug: Why reach out to other religions—even other denominations—when you were taught that your own had it all?

Even though I came late to the interfaith party, I was first introduced to yoga around 1970, through my much older half-brother. Richard was about thirty and I just twelve when he came to Maine to visit our shared father. In that Woodstock era Richard was encountering lots of new age folks for whom doing yoga was very hip. Richard didn't study with a guru but picked up enough hatha yoga and kundalini yoga from the people he met to form his own practice, and he even led a class for a time. I have a snapshot memory of our encounter, the image clear as a cloudless sky: Richard teaching me the lotus pose and a shoulder stand. I remember doing both at once, to our father's delight. The only other bit I recall was Richard's insistence that our father adopt a macrobiotic diet and chew each mouthful of brown rice fifty times. For our father it was a short-lived prescription, but the seed of curiosity about yoga that Richard planted in me would lay dormant for many decades before it began to germinate.

---

4. Charter for Compassion, accessed October 14, 2021, *https://charterforcompassion.org/*.

5. Karen Armstrong, *Twelve Steps to a Compassionate Life* (New York: Penguin, 2011).

Emerson and Thoreau: America's First Yogis

The yoga my hip half-brother Richard discovered for himself had lain slumbering in quiet corners of American life for over a century. In the 1840s at Walden Pond, Henry David Thoreau read the classic Hindu religious text the Bhagavad Gita and practiced some of the elements of yoga.[6] He was inspired by his good friend and contemporary, Ralph Waldo Emerson.

Trained as a Unitarian minister, Emerson served only briefly before becoming disenchanted with religious institutions. He felt Christian preaching had so downplayed the doctrine of God-within-us that it effectively buried the capacity of humans to manifest divine presence and creativity. In such preaching God was far away, and revelation was "something delivered once for all in the distant past [instead of] an immanent possibility."[7] What Emerson found lacking was the God-at-hand; the God who could be experienced alike by philosopher, laborer, and prisoner; the God of inspiration who pointed us to that better version of ourselves—the version God sees so clearly but that we often struggle to make out.

Emerson became a leader of transcendentalism, a philosophical movement that found unity in all creation, advocated for the intrinsic goodness of the human person, and gave weight to the validity of insight for discerning truth. Foundational to Emerson's teachings "was a vision of how every human being is, at depth, connected with the transcendental reality that infuses our universe with Law, Beauty, and Joy." He taught that God was radically immanent, universally available to the "properly attuned mind," and that "the only thing separating us from complete harmony with God's spiritual presence is a self-imposed, psychological barrier."[8]

Especially important was Emerson's assertion that Christian scriptures were not the sole repositories of truth and that some Eastern philosophies, such as Hinduism, set forth ideas that were superior to and filled in the gaps left by Western theology: "He championed Eastern religious ideas as a means of supplementing or complementing what our Western traditions offer, not as their antithesis."[9] Emerson brought ideas and language from Hindu mysticism into

---

6. Barbara Stoler Miller, "Why Did Thoreau Take the Bhagavad Gita to Walden Pond?" Yoga International, *https://yogainternational.com/article/view/why-did-thoreau-take-the-bhagavad-gita-to-walden-pond*, accessed September 29, 2021. For more information on Emerson and Thoreau as early yogis, see Stefani Syman, *The Subtle Body: The Story of Yoga in America* (New York: Farrar, Strauss, and Giroux, 2010).

7. Robert C. Fuller, *Spiritual but Not Religious: Understanding Unchurched America* (New York: Oxford University Press, 2001), 28.

8. Fuller, *Spiritual but Not Religious*, 28.

9. Fuller, *Spiritual but Not Religious*, 78.

mainstream in America. He died in 1882, and less than a decade later, the first Indian swami (monastic) would arrive in the United States.

Yoga Begins to Set Down Roots

Swami Vivekananda came from India in 1893 to speak at the Parliament of the World's Religions in Chicago, where he introduced the Hindu philosophy of Vedanta to a national audience. Arising as early as the sixth century BCE, Vedanta is the fertile ground from which yoga grew. Like Karen Armstrong would infer over a century later, Vivekananda proposed that the world's religions "are but various phases of one eternal religion."[10] They were paths, he declared, all leading to the same goal—union with the divine—and he made a compelling case that the similarities between religions far outnumbered their differences. His talk was enthusiastically received, as were the lectures he gave on a tour that followed the parliament.

Vivekananda spoke of "India's most sacred teaching: the divinity of man, his innate and eternal perfection; that this perfection is not a growth nor a gradual attainment, but a present reality. *That thou art.* You are that now. . . . We are not the helpless limited beings which we think ourselves to be, but birthless, deathless, glorious children of immortal bliss."[11] His teaching amplifies the words of Jesus: "You are the light of the world" (Matt. 5:14). Note the absence of any conditional language: not you *could be* or *will be* the light of the world, but you *are* the light of the world. You *are* a child of God. You *are* made in the divine image. To an audience likely taught that as descendants of Adam they came into the world stained by original sin and should thus scramble to avoid the wrath of a distant and angry God, Vivekananda's words had to be a comfort and a relief.

The next ambassador from India to make an impact was Paramahansa Yogananda, who traveled to Boston in 1920 as his country's delegate to the International Conference of Religious Liberals. Yogananda had founded a school in India to teach boys how to live.[12] His unique method combined academic teaching with yoga training and spiritual instruction. Yogananda spoke at the conference and was so warmly received that he spent the next fifteen years lecturing

10. Holly Hammond, "The Timeline and History of Yoga in America," *Yoga Journal*, August 28, 2007, *https://www.yogajournal.com/yoga-101/yogas-trip-america.*

11. Fuller, *Spiritual but Not Religious*, 81.

12. Self-Realization Fellowship, accessed October 14, 2021, *https://www.yogananda-srf.org/tmp/py.aspx?id=46&ekmensel=568fab5c_6_13_45_1.*

in the United States. In his talks, he "emphasized the underlying unity of the world's great religions, and taught universally applicable methods [specifically, yoga and meditation] for attaining direct personal experience of God."[13] In his later years, Yogananda focused his research and writing on the confluence of the Christian Gospels with yogic philosophy. The chance for "direct personal experience of God" would have been very appealing to Christians steeped in the doctrine of God's transcendence—so appealing, in fact, that he packed auditoriums from coast to coast. In Los Angeles, three thousand people filled a concert hall to capacity to hear his lecture, and thousands were turned away.[14]

Although Yogananda's lectures were warmly received, yoga didn't catch on widely at the time, inhibited in part by the 1924 Immigration Act. Driven by a fear that immigrants from Asia—including India—would work for substandard wages and steal American jobs and by a desire for racial homogeneity, the Act imposed quotas on Asian immigrants while giving preference to immigrants from Northern and Western Europe.[15]

Despite this, by the 1950s and 1960s, Americans were traveling to India to study yoga. Some returned home to open studios and teach yoga on television. A 1965 revision of US law removed the 1924 quota on Indian immigration,[16] and as a result more gurus were able to come from India to teach.

A yoga teacher from the Himalayas brought Transcendental Meditation to America in the early 1960s, books on yoga began to be published, ashrams opened, and some of the measurable health benefits of yoga began to be documented by the medical community. At the 1969 Woodstock Music Festival, when the arrival of the opening musical act was delayed by traffic, a kundalini yoga teacher took the stage and led the massive crowd through a simple class.[17] The Beatles' sojourn at an ashram in Rishikesh, India, for spiritual rejuvenation propelled yoga into the mainstream of American consciousness, as did former Harvard professor Ram Dass, poet Allen Ginsberg, and other countercultural voices of the Beat Generation of the 1950s and early 1960s.[18]

---

13. "A Beloved World Teacher," Self-Realization Fellowship, accessed October 14, 2021, *https://yogananda.org/a-beloved-world-teacher*.

14. "A Beloved World Teacher."

15. Richard Adler, "Immigration Act of 1924," Immigration to the United States, accessed October 14, 2021, *https://immigrationtounitedstates.org/590-immigration-act-of-1924.html*.

16. Lesley Kennedy, "How the Immigration Act of 1965 Changed the Face of America," History, August 12, 2019, *https://www.history.com/news/immigration-act-1965-changes*.

17. Gurujot Singh Khalsa, "Kundalini Yoga at Woodstock, Aug. 15, 1969!" Soul Answer, accessed October 14, 2021, *http://www.soulanswer.com/woodstock.html*.

18. Hammond, "The Timeline and History of Yoga in America."

Was It Something We Said?

In the Episcopal Church, the Rev. Alan Watts was on a search of his own for spiritual rejuvenation, and by 1950 he had left the church in pursuit of enlightenment in the Zen school of Buddhism and in the practice of yoga. Watts and others of the Beat Generation found the "doctrines and rituals that defined bourgeois American Christianity" to be "stultifying" and "hollow," and they searched for something that felt to them more spiritually pure. Like Emerson had before him, Watts rejected what he felt was the Church's "slavish worship of ancient dogmas" in favor of "nourish[ing his] own spiritual awakenings."[19]

Watts's letter of resignation from the priesthood, excerpted here, calls the church to release its grasp on doctrinal certainty and superiority:

> Insofar as the Church is committed to a desire for and a clinging to authority, permanence, spiritual safety, and absolute guides of conduct, it is clinging to its own death. By such means, belief in God, the hope of immortality, and the quest for salvation, become only escapes from the inner emptiness and insecurity which most of us feel in the depths of our being when confronted with the loneliness, the transiency, and the uncertainty of human life. But that inner emptiness is not a void to be filled with comforts; it is a window to be looked through. It is not an evil that life—our own life—flows, changes, and passes away. It is a revelation to prevent us from clinging to ourselves, for whoever lets go of himself finds God. The state of eternal life and oneness with God comes to pass—like a miracle—only when we release our grasp on every kind of spiritual security. To cling to security is only to cling to oneself, and perish of strangulation. . . .
>
> During the past years I have continued my studies of the spiritual teachings of the Orient, alongside with Catholic theology, and, though I have sometimes doubted it, I am now fully persuaded that the Church's claim to be the best of all ways to God is not only a mistake, but also a symptom of anxiety. Obviously, one who has found a great truth is eager to share it with others. But to insist—often in ignorance of other revelations—that one's own is supreme argues a certain inferiority complex characteristic of all imperialisms. . . . This claim of supremacy is, for me, the chiefest [*sic*] sign of how deeply the Church is committed to this self-strangulation, this anxiety for certainty, and I cannot support the proselytism in which it issues.[20]

---

19. Fuller, *Spiritual but Not Religious*, 28.

20. Alan Watts, *In My Own Way: An Autobiography* (Novato, CA: New World Library, 1972), 207–17.

Watts's call to be unafraid, to release clinging to that which seems to promise safety and security, and to self-empty is supported by the teaching of Jesus found in all four Gospels: "Those who find their life will lose it, and those who lose their life for my sake will find it" (Matt. 10:39). An echo of this teaching is found in the Upanishads: "So long as we remain exclusively attached to the outside world, we live in ignorance of our true spiritual nature."[21]

Some Episcopalians undoubtedly received Watts's writings as prophetic, prompting Christian leaders to feel a long-overdue humility. Indeed, his call to the Church would be picked up later by theologians such as Richard Rohr and Brian McLaren. Unfortunately, Watts's personal life and conduct did not befit a spiritual leader, and he and the Episcopal Church mutually took leave of each other. The importance of his message was discounted because the messenger was seen as so deeply flawed.

Despite the attention people like Watts and others brought to yoga as a worthwhile spiritual practice, in the 1960s yoga studios were sparse and, as one yoga teacher of the era put it, most "people confused yoga and yogurt. They were both brand new and nobody knew what either of them were."[22]

A surge of interest in physical fitness and spirituality in the 1970s helped yoga spread in the United States. Meanwhile, the Episcopal Church was introducing changes that not everyone embraced: the ordination of women, a new prayer book featuring more contemporary language, and a greater emphasis on the ministry of the laity. This likely contributed to the departure of hundreds of thousands of church members that was already well underway.

Or was this mass exodus caused by something else? It was more likely a disconnect between what we Christians said and how we lived—a limp that was visible to everyone except we who were walking. As Richard Rohr said, we told people what they should believe but failed to teach them how to live. We told them to pray, but we didn't teach them how or why. The elegant language of the prayers and collects in the Book of Common Prayer set a high bar and intimidated people from believing they could pray on their own. They thought a prayer had to be beautifully crafted to be pleasing or even acceptable to God. We told people to have faith but didn't give them a diverse collection of everyday tools they could use beyond Sundays to build and deepen a sense of union with the divine. The Daily Office (Morning Prayer, Noonday Prayer,

---

21. Fuller, *Spiritual but Not Religious*, 79.

22. Carolyn Gregoire, "How Yoga Became a $27 Billion Industry—and Reinvented American Spirituality," *HuffPost*, December 16, 2013, *https://www.huffpost.com/entry/how-the-yoga-industry-los_n_4441767*.

Evening Prayer, and Compline) was meant to be prayed by laypersons in their homes during the week, but it didn't allow people to *embody* their spirituality. We Episcopalians make a big deal of the physicality of the Incarnation, but our faith practices can often be rather heady.

People came to church looking for connection with God and for community with one another. They wanted to belong to something greater than themselves—something that gave them purpose and meaning. We proclaimed welcome and inclusiveness from the pulpit, but all too often our members failed to practice those values in the pews. Many Episcopal churches were places to "see and be seen," and while this country club atmosphere felt terrific to those on the inside, it was off-putting for those who were not.

I worked hard at St. John's, Boulder, to teach that hospitality and welcome are not merely attitudes but verbs, that acting hospitably is an actual spiritual practice. I was proud of my parish for embracing this teaching. I watched people carrying it out on Sunday mornings. But like any practice undertaken by human beings it is uneven: after Easter one year a man emailed me to tell me he was leaving the church. Again. It turns out he had been a parishioner before I arrived but left after feeling judged or alienated. He had heard I was a leader who truly seemed to care about welcoming everybody, so he came back to check things out. He attended for a couple months, and then, on Easter Sunday, had an experience that reopened his old wound.

Easter that year coincided with our monthly soup kitchen for those experiencing homelessness. On one end of the campus our three Easter morning services unfolded one after the other, while in the parish hall on the opposite side of the campus, a team of forty volunteers was gearing up to feed a hundred people and to offer basic medical care and haircuts. The man arrived to attend Easter worship. He was wearing jeans and a shirt. Stopping in the men's restroom, he stood at a urinal next to an older fellow in a blue blazer, crisp white shirt, and tie. The older man turned and looked at him, taking in his casual attire, and said, "These restrooms are for church members. The meal for the homeless is over there," as he nodded in the direction of the parish hall.

That is a disconnect between what we say we believe and how we live, and it is part of being imperfectly human. But it's good to remember that the crack between word and action is often wide enough to swallow up the timid seeker, who disappears, never to be seen in a pew again.

SBNR and the Appeal of Yoga

So where did all those church members go? Some stayed tucked into bed on Sunday mornings with a cup of coffee and the *New York Times*. Some read self-help books. Some remained affiliated with a church but only loosely so, attending worship services for Christmas, Easter, and perhaps a handful of other occasions. Some bounced from church to church and denomination to denomination. Others hauled their young children to church, hoping to implant in them a moral compass, but abandoned the effort when the already-overscheduled youngsters grew old enough to protest sitting in church while their soccer team was playing. A half-century ago, the world closed down on Sunday mornings in deference to churchgoers; not so today.

Many people who drifted away from regular church attendance joined the ranks of those who self-identify as "spiritual but not religious" (SBNR), a catch-all term so widely used that researchers have given it their attention and books have been devoted to its study. Robert C. Fuller, in *Spiritual but Not Religious: Understanding Unchurched America*, traces the history of this population and claims that "unchurched spirituality is gradually reshaping the faith of many who belong to mainstream religious organizations."[23] Surprisingly, 55 percent of all church members already hold private beliefs on the validity of spiritual practices well outside the bounds of the church's teachings.[24] The implications of the preceding two sentences cannot be understated.

If they are true, church leaders must learn not only who these SBNR folks are and what motivates them, but must also confront the fact that half the people presently sitting in our pews are drawing some of their beliefs from non-Christian sources and philosophies. We Episcopalians say that we are a church that "meets people where they are" and draws them into the faith. This seems to be where people are at this time in the church's history, and you can begin to see that these are populations for whom practicing yoga in a church would be appealing. A church considering offering yoga in its worship space needs to know something about their potential audience—both beyond the parish membership and within.

Fuller says that 90 percent of the US population claims to believe in a higher power, but nearly 40 percent of those have no enduring connection with organized religion.[25] Of that 40 percent, a quarter could be described as either

23. Fuller, *Spiritual but Not Religious*, 9.

24. Fuller, *Spiritual but Not Religious*, 9.

25. Fuller, *Spiritual but Not Religious*, 1.

(1) ambiguously religious, meaning that they attend more than six times a year but do not join the faith community; or (2) marginally religious, meaning that they join the community but attend less than six times a year.[26] In my parish, the ambiguously religious tend to sit in the back pews, may not choose to come forward to receive communion (despite the clergy's explicit and repeated invitation that all really are welcome), and often flee during the closing hymn so as to avoid the receiving line in the narthex. It is always a joy to me when they decide to take the leap and explore membership in the church. Regarding the marginally religious, in Episcopal lingo these are people often lovingly referred to as "C-and-E'ers"—Christmas and Easter attendees only.

Beyond the ambiguously and marginally religious are those who identify as spiritual but not religious. In 2001 Fuller estimated them to comprise as much as 21 percent of the American population. By 2017, their ranks had grown, comprising 27 percent of those surveyed by the Pew Research Center. Of that number, nearly half identified as having a Protestant or Roman Catholic affiliation but didn't identify strongly enough with a faith community to categorize themselves as "religious."[27]

Those who identify as SBNR draw from both traditional and nontraditional practices to create a framework of spiritual practice for themselves. They value intellectual freedom and curiosity and regard their lives as spiritual journeys whereon they look for regular insights and continual growth along the way. For them, the term *spiritual* is an adjective describing how a person understands themselves. "Religious" is how someone identifies publicly. They tend to see God (or the divine) as immanent and pervading all creation, making the entire universe a source of Spirit, and they believe that our true purpose is to be in harmony or union with this divine spirit.[28]

SBNR people tend to reject some of the tenets common in many expressions of institutional religion and presumed to be true by many of its adherents: biblical infallibility, a disregard for science or a subordination of science to faith, and a certainty that the institution has an exclusive hold on the truth. Philip Clayton of the Claremont School of Theology feels that while SBNR folks are not rejecting a sense of the divine, they do take issue

26. Fuller, *Spiritual but Not Religious*, 3.

27. Michael Lipka and Claire Gecewicz, "More Americans Now Say They're Spiritual but Not Religious," Pew Research Center, September 6, 2017, *https://www.pewresearch.org/fact-tank/2017/09/06/more-americans-now-say-theyre-spiritual-but-not-religious/*.

28. Fuller, *Spiritual but Not Religious*, 8.

with "religious organizations [being] too concerned with money and power, too focused on rules and too involved in the structures of the political status quo," and he calls for "a spirituality that is more open and accepting and evolutionary."[29]

Karen Hefford, a yoga teacher, musician, and Roman Catholic with a master's degree in theology, has spoken with many Christians about their experiences of yoga and what they find on the mat that is lacking for them in the pew. Those conversations reveal that through yoga, people learn to surrender, their spirituality feels embodied, and they are able to bring their personal experience to bear in communing with God. For some, yoga allows a gentle way to study the self, with all its shadows and contradictions. Hefford notes that people "have come to understand that they are so deeply flawed that the only way they can find love and comfort is from an external source."[30]

In our preaching and teaching have we focused too much on judgment and not enough on developing the doctrine of the unconditional and limitless love of God in Christ? It would appear so, and yet Scripture abounds with Jesus-loves-you-no-matter-what stories. In chapter 2, we'll take a look at how the Episcopal Church is well equipped to address the concerns of those who struggle with self-love and how those concerns can be addressed through the content of Yoga in the Church workshops.

It's not only the SBNR population that's lukewarm about institutional religion: Fuller cites research that indicates "a sizable percentage of church members have little loyalty to their churches' theological traditions"[31] and makes the point that the perspectives of church members and SBNR folks are often more alike than not. For such church members, their membership is more practical than affective, meaning that their involvement in the church depends heavily on the church's ability to educate their children and to provide their children and themselves with a sense of community, social contacts, and a feeling of meaning and purpose. When they find those lacking or absent, they disengage. In other words, the days when every parishioner was doggedly lifelong loyal to their denomination are rapidly disappearing.

---

29. "What Is Interspirituality?" On-Seeing, accessed October 14, 2021, *https://www.on-seeing.com/interspirituality.*

30. "About," Christ and Cascadia, accessed October 14, 2021, *http://www.journal.christandcascadia.com/about/.*

31. Fuller, *Spiritual but Not Religious*, 9.

The Enviable Growth of Yoga

Remember the parable of the mustard seed—how a little tiny seed inexplicably catapults into a big tree that provides essential shade from the relentless Middle Eastern sun? Yoga may well be one of the mustard seeds of our time. In recent years the growth of yoga practitioners in the United States has been nothing short of extraordinary.

Statistics on those who practiced yoga during the 1970s through early 2000s are sparse, although the circulation of *Yoga Journal* offers a hint: When it was founded in 1975, the magazine printed three hundred copies. Today, its total print readership is over 1.5 million.[32] The print circulation alone (not counting digital subscribers) of *Yoga Journal* is close to eclipsing the number of baptized Episcopalians (1,736,282).[33]

According to a 2008 study by *Yoga Journal*, 15.8 million Americans practiced yoga.[34] By 2012, that number had increased by 29 percent to 20.4 million,[35] and by 2016, 50 percent to 36 million.[36] The studies tend to cite flexibility, stress relief, and overall physical fitness and health as top motivators for a yoga practice. The 2016 Yoga in America study reported there were six thousand yoga studios operating in the United States, slightly less than the number of Episcopal parishes from that same time period—6,473.[37]

Thirty-six million people—that's more than ten times the Episcopal Church's membership in its best year. Are all these yoga practitioners finding God on their mats? Are they even searching? At first glance, not really. The 2016 Yoga in America study found that physical health and well-being (especially increasing one's strength, balance, and flexibility) and stress relief were top motivators for people who begin a practice of yoga. Despite this, a little more than 80 percent of yoga practitioners tend to agree that yoga is spiritual and has

32. Pocket Outdoor Media, "Yoga Journal Media Kit 2021," *https://images.saymedia-content.com/.image/cs_srgb/MTc2NDQ3Mjk2NTQyNjE0NzAx/yj-2021-media-kit.pdf, 9.*

33. The Episcopal Church, "The Episcopal Church: Baptized Members by Province and Diocese 2011-2020," *https://extranet.generalconvention.org/staff/files/download/30689*, 4.

34. Joelle Hann, "Yogi, Take Me to a Higher Place," *New York Times*, May 29, 2008, *https://www.nytimes.com/2008/05/29/health/nutrition/29fitness.html.*

35. YJ Editors, "New Study Finds More than 20 Million Yogis in U.S.," *Yoga Journal*, December 5, 2021, *https://www.yogajournal.com/blog/new-study-finds-20-million-yogis-u-s.*

36. Marilynn Wei, "New Survey Reveals the Rapid Rise of Yoga—and Why Some People Still Haven't Tried It," Harvard Health Publishing, March 7, 2016, *https://www.health.harvard.edu/blog/new-survey-reveals-the-rapid-rise-of-yoga-and-why-some-people-still-havent-tried-it-201603079179.*

37. The General Convention of the Episcopal Church, "Fast Facts: From Parochial Report Data 2020," *https://extranet.generalconvention.org/staff/files/download/30696.*

a role in a larger spiritual practice.[38] Even among nonpractitioners, around 60 percent believe that yoga is spiritual and has a place in spiritual practice.[39]

In studying who does yoga, other researchers have wondered "whether yoga attracts the spiritually inclined or whether yoga enhances spirituality" and suggest that future research explore the question more thoroughly.[40] Despite the dearth of statistical evidence, they do cite a 2009 study that found 67 percent of West Coast practitioners were motivated by "psychospiritual" reasons.[41] In an interview, Philip Goldberg, author of *American Veda*, articulated a connection between SBNR people and yoga practitioners, citing a common motivation for an individual to turn inward in order to connect with something beyond and larger than the self.[42]

Can the Episcopal Church—with our rich incarnational and mystical background—be an answer to this inclination? I believe so. In fact, as a Church, we (and other theologically broad-minded Christian denominations) are well equipped to offer yoga in our worship spaces, just as we do Centering Prayer, worship in the manner of Taizé, healing prayer, and labyrinth walks. It will take careful preparation and even a willingness to perhaps ruffle some feathers in the flock.

---

38. "2016 Yoga in America Study," Ipsos Public Affairs, January 2016, *https://www.yogaalliance.org/Portals/0/2016%20Yoga%20in%20America%20Study%20RESULTS.pdf, 26.*

39. "2016 Yoga in America Study," 42.

40. Crystal L. Park, Tosca Braun, and Tamar Siegel, "Who Practices Yoga? A Systematic Review of Demographic, Health-Related, and Psychosocial Factors Associated with Yoga Practice," *Journal of Behavioral Medicine* 38, no. 3 (January 2015): *https://www.researchgate.net/publication/271599510_Who_practices_yoga_A_systematic_review_of_demographic_health-related_and_psychosocial_factors_associated_with_yoga_practice.*

41. Park, Braun, and Siegel, "Who Practices Yoga?"

42. Gregoire, "How Yoga Became a $27 Billion Industry."

2

A THEOLOGICAL BASIS FOR THE COMPATIBILITY OF YOGA AND CHRISTIANITY

Do not fashion yourself in accordance with this material universe, but be spiritually re-made into something more excellent by the renovation and redecoration of the beautiful room of your intellect, so that then you might discern what is God's design and delight for you–all that is generous, well-pleasing; all that is full, whole, and complete.[1]

What Is Yoga?

To what exactly *are* we comparing the mystical, progressive Christian theology that is expressed by many Episcopal churches? Is yoga a religion or a philosophy? An exercise regime or a program of self-help? These definitions from leading yoga teachers and researchers, past and present, can help us understand what yoga is and what it is not:

> Yoga is an expansive discipline with profound philosophical reasoning that embraces the broad scope of human experience. At its core, it addresses the most fundamental need of the human being: to know one's spiritual self and to live in harmony with Spirit, in its absolute form (as spirit) as well as in creation.[2]

> Yoga, as a way of life and a philosophy, can be practiced by anyone with inclination to undertake it, for yoga belongs to humanity as a whole. It is not the property of any one group or any one individual, but can be followed by any and all, in any corner of the globe, regardless of class, creed or religion.[3]

1. The author's free translation of Romans 12:2 from the Greek.

2. Russill Paul, *Jesus in the Lotus: The Mystical Doorway between Christianity and Yogic Spirituality* (Novato, CA: New World Library, 2009), 8.

3. "K. Pattabhi Joise Quotes," AZ Quotes, accessed October 15, 2021, *https://www.azquotes.com/author/21798-K_Pattabhi_Jois.*

> Yoga is for internal cleansing, not external exercising. Yoga means true self-knowledge.[4]

> Yoga bridges different faiths and cultures "in the simplest of ways—by recognizing that God lives in each of us. . . . [I]n Biblical terms, 'bringing this mortal body to life through the Spirit dwelling within' is a pretty good description of how yoga works."[5]

> Yoga, an ancient but perfect science, deals with the evolution of humanity. This evolution includes all aspects of one's being, from bodily health to self-realization.

> Yoga restores to people, whatever religion they may belong to, the inner spiritual content [the "mystical core"] of their religion.[6]

> A yoga is a method—any one of many—by which an individual may become united with the Godhead, the Reality which underlies this apparent, ephemeral universe. To achieve such union is to reach the state of perfect yoga. Christianity has a corresponding term, "mystic union," which expresses a similar idea.[7]

> Yoga is the control of thought-waves in the mind.[8]

Kripalu Center for Yoga and Health, the school at which I trained for my 200-hour teacher certification, describes their particular stream of yoga as self-study with compassion. Founder Swami Kripalu observed that the highest spiritual practice is self-observation without judgment and that to perform every action artfully (mindfully—with intention, awareness, and care) is yoga. This practice of nonjudgmental observation is the way one is to regard the world as well.[9] Kripalu yoga offers the practitioner a way to harmonize the whole self—body, mind, and spirit—and to awaken compassionate awareness for oneself and one's world. (For a Christian, such compassionate awareness is an essential precondition to the practice of loving one's neighbor.) Yoga becomes a spiritual

---

4. "K. Pattabhi Joise Quotes."

5. Monette Chilson, *Sophia Rising: Awakening Your Sacred Wisdom through Yoga* (Houston: Bright Sky Press, 2013), 21–22.

6. Paul, *Jesus in the Lotus*, 12, quoting Swami Sivananda.

7. Swami Prabhavananda and Christopher Isherwood, trans., *How to Know God: The Yoga Aphorisms of Patanjali* (Hollywood, CA: Vedanta Press, 1953), 13.

8. Prabhavananda and Isherwood, trans., *How to Know God*, 14.

9. Kripalu 200-hour yoga teacher training, February 2020.

practice that, when done regularly, facilitates the process of transformation. Swami Kripalu likened God to the ocean and each of us as drops within that ocean.[10] Yoga is the meeting of Atman (the drop) and Brahman (the ocean), terms that are described in more detail later in this chapter.

In the Rig Veda, an ancient Indian religious text composed around 3000 BCE, *yoga* meant "chariot" or "journey," and drew on the root *yuj*, meaning to unite, yoke, or connect. If we think of the spiritual life as a journey—one on which we experience fleeting moments or even extended periods of such connection with God—that journey ends, finally, in unmitigated communion with the divine. Yoga is a tool that helps us make that journey. It's a journey Jesus invites us to embark on with him, saying, "Come to me, all you that are weary and are carrying heavy burdens, and I will give you rest. Take my yoke upon you and learn from me; for I am gentle and humble in heart, and you will find rest for your souls" (Matt. 11:28–29).

The Shortest Bridge Is between Yoga and Christianity's Wisdom and Mystical Traditions

Not long ago, my childhood best friend, Audrey, went through some long-unopened boxes of memorabilia from our school days. One thing she had stashed away was a hand-drawn card I had made for her and given to her in 1976 when we graduated from high school. On the front I had carefully calligraphed this Kahlil Gibran quotation: "When you reach the end of what you should know, you will be at the beginning of what you should sense."[11] I must have meant it as pithy life advice as we all prepared to leave for college and forge our way in the world. Writing in the introduction to his translation of the Upanishads, Eknath Easwaran says that "the world of the senses is just a base camp: we are meant to be as much at home in consciousness as in the world of physical reality."[12] What Gibran and Easwaran describe is where the church needs to stand right now as we nose our way forward into an unmapped future. We need to set aside our intellectual knowing and have the courage and faith to "know" with our hearts.

Russill Paul declares that Christianity has so domesticated God that the church has all but lost the "cosmic dimension of religious experience." He

10. Kripalu 200-hour yoga teacher training, February 2020.

11. *https://www.goodreads.com/quotes/21605-when-you-reach-the-end-of-what-you-should-know.*

12. *The Upanishads*, introduced by and trans. Eknath Easwaran (Tomales, CA: Nilgiri Press, 1987), 10.

points us back to the medieval Christian mystics and to the ancient Celtic expression of Christianity to recapture a sense of vastness and mystery and to restore our balance. He urges us to focus less on salvation and more on wisdom so that we might recover the depth of our tradition and "relate meaningfully to the Eastern wisdom-based traditions such as yoga."[13]

In her book *The Wisdom Jesus*, Cynthia Bourgeault, Episcopal priest and contemporary theologian in the wisdom tradition, speaks of Jesus

> first and foremost as a wisdom teacher, a person who . . . clearly emerges out of and works within an ancient tradition called "wisdom," sometimes known as *sophia perennis*, which is in fact at the headwaters of all the great religious traditions of the world today. It's concerned with the transformation of the whole human being. Transformation from what to what? Well, for a starter, from our animal instincts and egocentricity into love and compassion; from a judgmental and dualistic worldview into a nondual acceptingness.[14]

This isn't to negate or even downplay Jesus as the incarnation of God, second person of the Trinity, or as our prayer book says, "the author of our salvation."[15] This depiction of Jesus as wisdom teacher is to augment other descriptions of him, and as wisdom teacher he stands closer to yogic philosophy than he does perhaps in his other roles.

The wisdom and mystical traditions are part of Christianity but transcend it and, as Bourgeault says, can be found at the headwaters of all the great religious traditions of the world. In Christianity, at least, over the centuries Enlightenment thinking gradually supplanted mysticism, once the birthright of all believers.

Perhaps (likely) I wasn't paying attention, or perhaps those who taught me were not taught this themselves (also likely) so didn't know to pass it on, but growing up in the Episcopal Church I wasn't exposed to the mystical dimension of my faith. I was taught to regard Jesus primarily as Savior—someone who had and would continue to rescue me from my badness. I also was taught that because of his goodness and my badness and unworthiness, he was necessary to serve as the personal delivery boy of my prayers to God. He was someone I was supposed to admire and emulate, but the idea that he and I could converse as

---

13. Paul, *Jesus in the Lotus*, 6.

14. Cynthia Borgeault, *The Wisdom Jesus: Transforming Heart and Mind—A New Perspective on Christ and His Message* (Boston: Shambala Publications, 2008), 4.

15. *The Book of Common Prayer* (New York: Church Hymnal Corporation, 1979), 369.

friends was never a concept to which I was introduced. To hear that that is one of the whole points of the gospel was news to me.

Knowing now that such union is not only possible, but that God actually intends and longs for us to enjoy this union, I can reflect on my life and identify many moments that would qualify as mystical. As a child and young adult, without definition, frame of reference, or permission, I thought mystical experience of God was the exclusive property of monks and nuns and could therefore never be mine.

Contemporary mystical theologian Richard Rohr, writing for the Center for Action and Contemplation, says that "a mystic is simply *one who has moved from mere belief or belonging systems to actual inner experience of God.* Mysticism is more represented in John's gospel than in the other three gospels, which tend to give us the basic story line of Jesus' life, death, and resurrection. Perhaps many readers are not moved by or attracted to John's gospel because they were never taught the mystical mind."[16]

Had I been "taught the mystical mind" in my formative years, my life would have felt more tethered to something sacred, something larger and beyond myself. The Christian institution is failing its youth when we don't help them claim their birthright as mystics. And we wonder why they drift away from church. Rohr points back to Karl Rahner, influencer of Vatican II, who said that "if Western Christianity does not discover its mystical foundations and roots, we might as well close the church doors." Rohr adds that "without a contemplative mind, Christianity can't offer broad seeing, real alternative consciousness, or a new kind of humanity. Jesus was the first clear nondual mystic in the West. . . . We just were not prepared for his way of knowing and loving."[17]

What distinguishes Christian mysticism, says Rohr, is that it is incarnational, and we need to reclaim this as our essential theme and specialty. In the Incarnation, God "said yes to all that was physical, material, and earthly." Rohr explains that

> until people have had some *mystical, inner spiritual experience,* there is no point in asking them to follow the ethical ideals of Jesus or to really understand religious beliefs beyond the level of formula. At most, such moral ideals and doctrinal affirmations are only a source of deeper anxiety because we don't have the power to follow any of Jesus' major teachings about forgiveness,

16. Richard Rohr, "Incarnational Mysticism," Center for Action and Contemplation, July 14, 2019, *https://cac.org/incarnational-mysticism-2019-07-14/.*

17. Rohr, "Incarnational Mysticism."

> love of enemies, nonviolence, humble use of power, a simple lifestyle, and so on, except in and through radical union with God.[18]

To have power, he concludes, doctrines have to be experienced and not merely ascribed to with the rational mind. Or, as I wrote to Audrey in her graduation card, we must move from the end of what we should know to the beginning of what we should sense. This is the space where yoga and Christianity can meet charitably.

Imagine a high-arched bridge over a wide and beautiful river that is the border between two countries. The water's surface glitters in the sun. As you stand on the bank of your homeland, you can see the other country on the other side. But you have no spotting scope, no binoculars, so you can't make out any details. For all you know the flowers might emit different fragrances there; the wind might sound different as it moves through the trees; the people might look and speak quite differently from you. As you stand on your bank, another soul stands on the opposite shore, on the bank of the place he was born and raised, the place he will always call home, the place where one day his body will rest according to the burial customs of his people.

You and he step onto the bridge from your opposite sides. You both ascend higher and higher until you meet in the highest place—the middle. The view from there is loftier than anything you've ever seen. You are seeing, you think, as an eagle sees. You can see your land, its buildings and roads and people, its industry and agriculture, its weather systems forming and dissipating over distant ranges. You can see these same features in the land of your new friend.

You bow toward each other in greeting. There is a bench, and you sit a while. You each talk, and you each listen with a relaxed curiosity. You each note delightful similarities in your respective cultures as well as stark differences. There is no competition as to whose is better. There is no pressure to press the two into one mold. The sun falls from its apex into the western sky, appearing to sink more rapidly as it nears the horizon. It is the same sun that enlivens and sustains you both. The shadows lengthen. It is time to go. You both laugh because although you are each of modest stature, the sun has made you cast shadows long as beans. You choose to embrace for your farewell because each of you is more than you were when you ascended the bridge. You and your new friend each return to your home countries, happy to be who you are and where you live but changed forever by the encounter,

18. Rohr, "Incarnational Mysticism."

and knowing you will go to the place of meeting again and again, where both of you will learn.

A charitable meeting place.

What Impedes Us from Moving to the Center of This Bridge Where Yoga and Christianity May Meet?

A conception of yoga as a religion can lead good, traditional Episcopalians to be suspicious of it, fearful that practicing yoga sets one on a slide into idolatry. You don't need more than a passing acquaintance with the Bible to be reminded that the warnings against idolatry are numerous, the story of the golden calf in Exodus 32 being perhaps the best known.

According to the Epistles, the early Christians had their hands full trying to spread the gospel through a Greco-Roman world where fertility cults and civic religions that worshipped idols were pervasive. In his first letter to the Corinthians (8:4b–6), Paul says,

> we know that "no idol in the world really exists," and that "there is no God but one." Indeed, even though there may be so-called gods in heaven or on earth—as in fact there are many gods and many lords—yet for us there is one God, the Father, from whom are all things and for whom we exist, and one Lord, Jesus Christ, through whom are all things and through whom we exist."

We are a denomination for whom Holy Scripture and tradition are important and cherished ways we understand and express our faith, and anything that scratches too deeply into that mortar is suspect. I can sympathize: visit some yoga studios, and you'll encounter unfamiliar statues or art. You might see Hindu gods such as Shiva, sitting in a lotus position and representing liberation and freedom, gained through the destruction of old unhelpful habits and ego-feeding ways; Ganesh, Shiva's son, the elephant-headed god who helps one remove obstacles that impede success; Lakshmi, the feminine goddess of light, beauty, and good fortune; and Lord Hanuman, the monkey god, who embodies devotion and courage.

It's important to know that Hindus do not regard themselves as polytheists but as pluralists, seeing these (and other) gods as diverse manifestations and expressions of the one reality, God—Brahman—whose image is unknowable. In contrast, Christians regard Jesus Christ as the primary manifestation, expression, and incarnation of the Lord God, whose image, like that of Brahman, is unknowable. Many progressive Christians see creation—both its animate and inanimate aspects—as another manifestation of God, perhaps even the *first* incarnation of God. After all, creation begins with God's most intimate outpouring: the divine breath.[19]

Many yoga studios don't emphasize Hindu gods or philosophy at all, substituting terms like *energy*, *life force*, and *spirit* to explain the relationship between humanity and creation. There is no statue, icon, or art that is essential to the practice of yoga, and no worship nor acknowledgment of deities of any kind is necessary. If desired, a simple flower and a candle can suffice to draw the attention beyond oneself toward the peace that passes understanding, the peace that underlies the cosmos.

So, *is* yoga a religion? Is it synonymous with Hinduism, and does bringing yoga into the church threaten to make us Episco-Hindus? These questions are not to be taken lightly, and the question of whether yoga is a religion is a question the courts have addressed. In a 2013 case brought by California parents concerned about yoga being taught in schools, the school district (the defendant in the case)

> contracted two scholars of Indian religion and specifically of Hindu yogic traditions. Dr. Mark Singleton, a senior researcher at the School of Oriental and African Studies in London and an expert in the history of modern yoga, particularly its permutations in India in the last 150 years and its transition to the US through the influence of various *gurus*, testified that yoga as it is practiced today in the US was "a distinctly American cultural phenomenon . . . rooted in American culture as much (and sometimes far more) than in Indian culture."
>
> The second expert witness hired by the defendants, Dr. Chris Chapple, a professor of theology at Loyola Marymount University and an expert on Indian yogic traditions, testified that yoga, even if it were to be considered religious, is not confined by any single religion, but practiced by people of almost all religions and of no religion at all. Yoga, in Chapple's testimony, appears as a device of practice, the content of which, religious or not, is supplied by the practitioner.[20]

---

19. Genesis 1:2 says, "The Spirit of God hovers over the waters." Another translation of "spirit" is "breath." The New Analytical Greek Lexicon, Wesley J. Perschbacher, Ed., Peabody, MA: Hendrickson Publishers, 1990, 334, Strong's Concordance #4151.

20. Sunila S. Kale and Christian Lee Novetzke, "Yoga and the Means and Ends of Secularism," The Wire, June 21, 2018, ***https://thewire.in/government/yoga-means-ends-secularism.***

In essence, the ruling, upheld by an appellate court of appeal, was that yoga is both religious and nonreligious, depending on how it's engaged. The appellate court explained that "a reasonable observer would not conclude that an activity has the primary effect of advancing religion merely because of its historical association with religion."[21] Yoga certainly has strong religious roots, and yet its Westernization has often completely ignored those roots, to the dismay and even anger of Hindus. It is possible to practice yoga and subscribe to Hindu rituals and beliefs. It is also possible to practice yoga and harvest only its mind and body calming and focusing techniques. And it is possible to harvest those techniques and greet the attendant beliefs with curiosity as to what they might say about God in whom Christians live and move and have their being. Being able to articulate this point will help Episcopal clergy and lay leaders seeking to introduce yoga to their parishes.

Historically, while yoga has always had a strong connection to spirituality in the context of religion, it came into being on its own, apart from Hinduism and Buddhism. Like these two faith traditions, yoga was born in the ancient pre-Hinduism, pre-Buddhism Vedic culture of the Indian subcontinent. Eknath Easwaran believes the beginnings of yoga may have occurred in northern India, in the Indus River valley, and roughly coincided with the building of the Egyptian pyramids along the Nile, perhaps 3,000 years before the birth of Christ. He cites the discovery of an image of Shiva as *Yogeshvara* (the Lord of yoga) as evidence to "suggest that meditation was practiced in a civilization which flourished a millennium before the Vedas [pre-Hindu religious texts] were committed to an oral tradition."[22]

Vedic scholar David Frawley notes that while yoga does not insist one hold a certain belief system, much of classical yoga philosophy nonetheless includes teachings—such as karma and rebirth—that are at odds with Christian doctrine.[23] My sense is that on the surface, such teachings are indeed opposed to Christian teachings, and when introducing yoga to a church we need to be frank about that. But if one looks beneath the surface of both yogic philosophy and Christianity, perhaps our doctrines are pointing to the same things, the same values, the same human longing for union with God.

I believe that we can engage yoga in the church without hybridizing our faith and without collapsing the great religious traditions of Christianity and

---

21. Kale and Novetzke, "Yoga and the Means and Ends of Secularism."

22. *The Bhagavad Gita*, introduced by and trans. Eknath Easwaran (Tomales, CA: Nilgiri Press, 2007), 16.

23. Andrea Ferretti, "Yoga as a Religion?," *Yoga Journal*, March 1, 2012, *https://www.yogajournal.com/yoga-101/beyond-belief*.

Hinduism into one. True to my Episcopalian heritage, I propose a middle way that honors the importance of human reason to this matter. Here's the litmus test for me: Can this practice or philosophy help me better understand and more deeply and richly live my Christian faith, or does it denigrate it and seek to draw me from it? We follow a boundary-breaking Lord, and yet we are quick to fence in our faith tradition and protect its "purity" by calling it *orthodoxy*. If we are consumed with worry about stepping outside the bounds of our faith, it surely cannot be because we feel Jesus needs our protection! More likely it's because we know and interact too little with people of other monotheistic religions and so assume they have nothing to offer us.

In 2007 while on summer break from seminary, I interned at St. John's Cathedral in Denver and became involved with The Abrahamic Initiative there. The initiative brought Jews, Muslims, and Christians together in small groups over a shared meal. People didn't talk about the doctrines of their respective religions as much as they talked about their dreams, their struggles, and their kids. As I got to know an imam, I began to uncover and soften my well-hidden bias against people who didn't worship from the Book of Common Prayer.

That relatively brief summer of interfaith dialogue opened my eyes to what might be called an interspiritual landscape of reality. Brother Wayne Teasdale was one of the first to speak of interspirituality, and as a monastic in both the Roman Catholic and Hindu traditions, he lived what he taught. Interspirituality has been defined as

> that deeper unity of experience that is our shared spiritual heritage, irrespective of our outer religion or lack thereof. It is the common ground—the fountainhead—which lies beneath the diversity of theological beliefs, rites, and observances. Interspirituality sees this mystical spirituality as the origin of all the world religions, and posits that every authentic spiritual path offers unique perspectives and rich insights into this deeper, direct experience of truth.[24]

Interspirituality has been called "the common ground, where all of the wisdom traditions meet"[25] or, as Bourgeault put it, "the headwaters."

Interspirituality is not the same as syncretism. In seminary, the evils of syncretism were painstakingly laid out for me, illustrated by all the heresies of

---

24. "What Is Interspirituality?"

25. Joan Borysenko, "What Is Interspirituality?," Joan Borysenko, PhD, accessed October 15, 2021, *https://www.joanborysenko.com/spirituality/what-is-interspirituality/*.

the early church. Ancient Christian theology must have been like taffy, being continuously pulled, stretched, drooped, and looped back upon itself. And yet, heresies aside, the early church was still deeply shaped by Judaism and Hellenism. So, in some respects, it came out of the gate already somewhat syncretized. Beyond that, true religious syncretism, simply put, is the melting together of two religions so thoroughly that each one loses its original identity. Melt some red crayons and some blue ones together, and good luck trying to separate the purple slurry back into two distinct colors. Interspirituality is more of a tossed salad, wherein the avocado, the heirloom tomatoes, and the leftover grilled corn all complement each other and create something together that each could not be on its own, with one important distinction: the avocado doesn't lose its avocado-ness; the heirloom tomato doesn't sacrifice its tomato-ness; the grilled kernels of corn do not give up their corn-ness.

Religious syncretism is not at all what Yoga in the Church is about. We respect the distinct cultural contexts in which Hinduism and Christianity arose. We see them as two equally honorable and fully standalone faith traditions. We acknowledge that many of their doctrines may parallel in appealing and mutually instructive ways, but there are many, many teachings, practices, and beliefs where the two traditions diverge. We do not seek to make them agree. We use yoga's philosophical insights and practices as tools to delve deeper into Christian faith, and we pray that the places where yogic philosophy and progressive, mystical Christian theology say the same thing become sparks that ignite people's curiosity about the Christian faith.

This approach sets Yoga in the Church apart from certain other streams of "Christian yoga." One Christian yoga school embraces breath work (pranayama), meditation, and asanas (postures) but encourages teachers to use English terms instead of Sanskrit so there's no risk that practitioners will think they're endorsing Hinduism.[26] The school rejects any discussion of chakras (energy centers in the body) or the chanting of "Om" or "Aum," the universal sound of the divine. Some Christian practitioners relabel asanas with more Christian-sounding names. For example, a sun salutation might become a Son salutation so there is no doubt in anyone's mind that the practice is being dedicated to the Son of God—Jesus Christ.[27] Another school bills its fitness movements as the Christian alternative to yoga and counsels that while pranayama

26. "What We Believe," Holy Yoga, accessed October 15, 2021, *https://holyyoga.net/about/what-we-believe/*.

27. "Christoga—Christian Yoga," YouTube video, 1:18, September 14, 2007, *https://www.youtube.com/watch?time_continue=76&v=PpcYPiE6A1s&feature=emb_logo*.

may be pleasantly and temporarily mind-numbing, it is a dangerous gateway to the new age and is no substitute for the peace Paul describes in Philippians 4:7—the peace which passes understanding.[28] (Personally, I think God's peace is more than expansive and universal enough to be accessed by pranayama as well as more orthodox forms of Christian prayer.)

In our workshops we speak of the places that yogic philosophy and Christian theology and scripture point to the same things, and we also speak of the places where they do not. Our goal is to convert no one but simply to deepen the faith of all, whatever their faith may be. If someone becomes a Christian because of Yoga in the Church, they do so because we have provided them a gentle doorway through which they can respond to the invitation of God. One group that appears to share our approach is christianspracticingyoga.com. Their website content reflects a respect for the standalone integrity of both Eastern philosophy and Western Christian theology:

> We are an organization [whose members include Baptists, Roman Catholics, Episcopalians, Lutherans, Methodists, Eastern Orthodox, Presbyterians, United Church of Christ, and many others] that studies the intersections of yoga philosophy and Christian theology—and the practices of both—in order to provide support, education, and community for an interdenominational Christian audience. . . . We envision a time when, through the deep transformative power of Christ, Christians practicing yoga and contemplative prayer make a significant contribution to healing the divides in our lives and in our world.[29]

The Way-Finders

The discussion of moving to a meeting place would not be complete without a mention of some of those pioneering souls who ascended the bridge before us and who have returned there again and again. They show us the way. It's often the voices of those who've been relegated to the edges of orthodoxy that are in the best position to break away from the pack and show us something interesting—to offer us a new way of seeing.

Fr. Jean-Marie Déchanet, a Benedictine priest serving in the Congo and later in France, wrote a book called *Christian Yoga*, first published in French,

---

28. "The Dangers of Yoga," Praise Moves, accessed October 15, 2021, *https://praisemoves.com/about-praisemoves/why-a-christian-alternative-to-yoga/the-dangers-of-yoga/.*

29. Chrisitians Practicing Yoga, "Our Mission," *https://www.christianspracticingyoga.com/our-mission.*

in 1956. In it he argued that Christians can benefit from practicing yoga, especially since Western Christians live in a noisy, turbulent world, and it is only in inner stillness that God can be heard. Yoga, he felt, was a tool to move us toward that stillness. Déchanet studied the work of the twelfth-century mystic William of Saint-Thierry and was particularly drawn to Saint-Thierry's assertion that three principles of activity in a human person had to be in balance with one another as a precondition for experiencing union with God. Saint-Thierry identified those three principles as (1) *anima*, or the life of the body and its functions; (2) *animus*, or the conscious, thinking, reasoning intellect; and (3) *spiritus*, or that within us that moves us toward love, toward beauty, toward the good, toward God.[30]

After Déchanet read an article about yoga, he realized its usefulness to help bring the three aspects into balance, achieving the necessary precondition for experiencing union with God. It was this union that was always Déchanet's goal. He understood that as he worked toward achieving this balance, God would extend to him grace. He and God would be reaching toward each other.

Déchanet wrote:

> It is a harmony among these "three" [anima, animus, and spiritus] that is sought in each of us by the grace of redemption. Christ came in the first place so that this "creature of God" within us, concealed under a human complex, bruised and torn by original sin, should flower and open out in its full beauty and wealth of talent. Any ascetic discipline that works towards this works, in fact, hand in hand with grace, and that is why I have roundly stated that a yoga that calms the senses, pacifies the soul, and frees certain intuitive or affective powers in us can be of inestimable service to the West. It can make people into true Christians, dynamic and open, by helping them to be men.[31]

Déchanet was extremely careful not to collapse yoga and Christianity together into one. He drew from yoga those elements that served to deepen his Christian spiritual practices such as contemplative prayer. He worried that Europeans were ignoring the spiritual aspects of yoga, whittling it down to the physical postures so that for them it became little more than a sport.[32] Déchanet had some support from his superiors in the church, and yet he was not without his detractors. The altered state of mind brought about by slow,

30. Jean-Marie Déchanet, OSB, *Christian Yoga* (London: Search Press, 1960), 64–65.

31. Déchanet, *Christian Yoga*, 12–13.

32. Déchanet, *Christian Yoga*, 31.

measured asanas and breathing exercises (pranayama) that Déchanet found such a useful catalyst to contemplative prayer was cast as the devil's playground by other Catholics who felt that such a state of mind opened one to demonic influence.[33]

Father Bede Griffiths was another pioneer of the interspiritual movement, living a rich and scholarly life at Shantivanam, a Benedictine monastery–ashram in South India. As a young man, Griffiths excelled at Oxford, became friends with C. S. Lewis, and sought ordination in the Church of England. Church officials advised Griffiths that before he pursued the priesthood he should first go get some real-life experience. Griffiths was discouraged and deeply confused. He lost himself in prayer and eventually found a home in Roman Catholicism. As a Roman Catholic priest, Griffiths discovered yoga and ancient Indian religious texts through a colleague before heading to India in the mid-1950s.

Eventually, under his leadership, Shantivanam established a reputation as a place to learn and practice the contemplative life and to learn from a religion other than one's own.[34] The monks and seekers there followed the Rule of St. Benedict and studied Hindu religious texts and philosophy. They practiced yoga as a way of moving deeper into prayer and contemplation. At the monastery, Griffiths blended Christian and Hindu imagery, movement, chanting, meditation, and prayer into a unique interspiritual liturgy that included the celebration of Holy Eucharist. In the words of Russill Paul, one the former monks there, the eucharistic liturgy felt "authentically Christian, yet authentically Hindu."[35] He felt an energy underlying the liturgy that drew him almost effortlessly into the mystery of Christ. For Paul, the Eucharist is a twofold act of thanksgiving in which we offer our gratitude for God's interest in our welfare and our appreciation for God's "invitation to participate at the core of the Divine life."[36] It is a public ritual whose effect is nonetheless intensely personal, as the worshiper engages in "loving reciprocity" and relationship building with God.

In his book *Jesus in the Lotus*, Paul writes, "It was Bede Griffiths's genius not only to reconcile Christianity and Hinduism but also to do so in a way that created a harmonious whole utterly respectful of both parts. . . . Bede was

---

33. Brother Max Sculley, DLS, "Dechanet's Christian Yoga," Brother Max Sculley, accessed October 15, 2021, *http://maxsculley.blogspot.com/2013/07/dechanets-christian-yoga.html*.

34. Pascaline Coff, OSB, "Man, Monk, Mystic," Bede Griffiths, accessed October 15, 2021, *http://www.bedegriffiths.com/man-monk-mystic/*.

35. Paul, *Jesus in the Lotus*, 90.

36. Paul, *Jesus in the Lotus*, 87.

critical of the idea that you can use established traditions as if they were bins of raw materials from which to randomly select parts for assembling a religious practice."[37] As Paul responded to the call from God to the life of a Benedictine monk at Shantivanam (and later, to life as a married Christian), he himself became something of a bridge between the Hindu faith of his ancestors and the Christian faith to which he was called.

Paul suggests that Christianity and yoga actually complement and complete each other. Yoga's emphasis on the practitioner's striving to meet God can benefit from the Christian perspective that God is an eternal outpouring of love and grace on all that God has made. In other words, Christianity can offer yoga a God who makes an effort to meet us just as we make an effort to meet God.[38] Christianity also offers a social dimension to love. While yoga primarily addresses the loving relationship between the seeker and the divine, Christianity and Judaism both call the individual to extend that love to others. God blesses us, *and* we are to be a blessing to others (Gen. 12:2). Paul says that "the practice of love is a Yoga in itself, and . . . Christians are arguably the masters of it, or so they should be."[39]

Paul argues that the power of Christlike love transforms not only the lover but the one loved: "The Yoga of Jesus is to love, despite the other's ego, despite their karma, despite their ignorance, for the power of love can transform their ego and their karma and their ignorance."[40] This transformation is a process that happens over time, and its social dimension—in other words, the power of one person's love to be transformative for others—is what Christianity can contribute to "the communal process of enlightenment."[41]

This enlightenment, says Paul, is a gradual, participatory, individual, communal, and societal process that involves the entire creation and calls Christ to the present. Instead of Jesus Christ's Second Coming being an event, it is a cosmos-wide process: "The Second Coming of Jesus is better seen as a gradual process that ushers in a new consciousness, a process that requires our consent and conscious participation."[42] I find this a refreshing alternative to the biblical depiction of the Son of Man coming without warning (or prefaced by

---

37. Paul, *Jesus in the Lotus*, 70–71.

38. Paul, *Jesus in the Lotus*, 164.

39. Paul, *Jesus in the Lotus*, 166.

40. Paul, *Jesus in the Lotus*, 170.

41. Paul, *Jesus in the Lotus*, 171.

42. Paul, *Jesus in the Lotus*, 172.

apocalyptic signs that no one's been able to figure out for millennia) on roiling clouds; like a thief in the night; attended by trumpets, saints, and angels; landing somewhere in the Middle East; ready to judge the unsuspecting peoples of the earth. Such a depiction has always called to mind for me the image of a divine military parade, lacking only the tanks and missile launchers. Wouldn't it better suit the Lord of Love to come as a gradual and inclusive awakening?[43]

Harvard divinity professor Francis X. Clooney is a scholar of Hindu-Christian studies who suggests that Patanjali's Yoga Sutras may be studied together with Ignatius of Loyola's *Spiritual Exercises*. Like others who show us the way, Clooney acknowledges that yoga and Christianity have real theological differences. Further, because they are grounded in two very different cultures, each lacks the vocabulary to do justice to the other.[44] Nonetheless, he finds the conclusion of the Yoga Sutras (4.29–34) and the conclusion of the *Spiritual Exercises* to both point to the same state of being: "a person who sees the world as a whole, as it were God who sees it, who has received all by grace, who acts only in utter freedom . . . detached, free, at peace, acting without need."[45] Like Russill Paul, Clooney sees yoga and Christianity (specifically, Ignatian spirituality) as complementary:

> The Ignatian ideal infuses yoga with a language of love, and Patañjali's ideal infuses the Exercises with a fuller sense of the utter simplicity and freedom of seeing the world serenely, all at once. (And still, a simpler possibility remains: yoga can teach a practitioner of the Exercises how to give herself in love more serenely and freely, while the Exercises can teach yoga practitioners how to imagine a person, the Person, in whom the world reaches peace and becomes a gift again.)[46]

Launched in 2016, Ignatian yoga is a Jesuit-endorsed program that combines Ignatian spirituality and yogic philosophy and practices. Their aim is not to use asanas and pranayama solely as a means to deeper prayer, but to bring Christian theology and yogic philosophy into culturally sensitive and

---

43. Those curious to learn more about the awakening of consciousness as the gradual coming of Christ could study the work of twentieth-century French Jesuit paleontologist and mystic Pierre Teilhard de Chardin and an interpretation of his work on this topic by Ilia Delio, OSF, Christ in Evolution (Maryknoll, NY: Orbis Books, 2008).

44. Francis X. Clooney, SJ, "Jesuit Yoga: The Finale," *America: The Jesuit Review*, August 8, 2008, *https://www.americamagazine.org/content/all-things/jesuit-yoga-finale*.

45. Clooney, "Jesuit Yoga: The Finale."

46. Clooney, "Jesuit Yoga: The Finale."

respectful conversation with each other. In this, their mission is similar to that of Yoga in the Church.[47]

In the Episcopal Church, Nancy Roth was among the first to advocate for the place of yoga in the life of the Christian. In the 1970s she took a yoga class and found it helped her connect her own embodied humanity and divinity with that of Jesus Christ. She found yoga conducive to Christian prayer and didn't regard the chanting of "Om" or the Sanskrit names for asanas to be stumbling blocks. In her 2005 book, *An Invitation to Christian Yoga*, Roth explained how to link certain basic asanas with biblical verses or lines of prayers to enable the practitioner to engage the body in worshiping God.

In Texas, Episcopal priest the Rev. Gena Davis has, like Bede Griffiths, woven together the celebration of Holy Eucharist with meditation, yogic breath work, and asanas, aiming to deepen the experience of the sacrament and better equip worshipers to open the heart, the body, and the intellect to Christ in new and deeper ways. It is beyond the present scope of Yoga in the Church to offer the sacrament of Communion to yogic practitioners as part of our classes. To be done responsibly, it requires additional layers of teaching and preparation for both the parish and the practitioners. For those curious to learn more, Davis's book *YogaMass: Embodying Christ Consciousness* is a helpful resource.

Our Uneasy Relationship with the Human Body

The last hurdle to bringing yoga into the church undoubtedly deserves a book of its own. Our uneasy relationship with the human body is an issue that extends beyond the Episcopal Church and endures in the Episcopal Church despite our self-identification as progressive. What a paradox that we who scandalously believe that human flesh was good enough for God to come and dwell therein have historically minimized or ignored the importance of not only caring for that body, that divine container, but of actually using it to encounter God.

We speak of "embodied faith" and Jesus, our *embodied* Lord—God in human flesh. Our faith rests on bodily events: the birth, crucifixion, and resurrection of the body and person of Jesus. Jesus's bodily humanity is what makes his relevance for us so believable and powerful. In the Holy Eucharist, our principal sacrament, we repeat Jesus's own words, "This is my *body*, given for you."

47. Joe Hoover, SJ, "What's the Deal with Ignatian Yoga? A Skeptical Jesuit Finds Out," America: The Jesuit Review, February 8, 2019, *https://www.americamagazine.org/faith/2019/02/08/whats-deal-ignatian-yoga-skeptical-jesuit-finds-out-232548.*

When I am the celebrant, I inevitably emphasize that word, because for me the wonder of his gift is ever new. In speaking of the church, we echo Paul, who spoke of the *ecclesia* as Christ's body. At Episcopal funerals, the priest opens the service by singing or saying an anthem that evokes Job 19: "After my awaking he will raise me up and *in my body* I shall see God."[48]

Even so, Christians have downplayed the potential for the human body to be an altar where we greet and worship God. We miss the opportunity to respond to the Eucharist by saying back to Jesus, "And this is *my* body, dear Lord, given for *you*!" Russill Paul says that yoga recognizes that a practitioner's "most powerful and sacred vessel of Self-realization" (i.e., realizing the God within us) is their human body, and adds that "yoga can help to integrate the body and its processes more intimately in prayer experience."[49]

I agree with Paul that "Christianity has become predominantly a thinking religion."[50] The Episcopal Church, with our fondness for meeting God through the intellect, is especially at risk of dismissing the importance of meeting God through the body and through the heart as well.

At Kripalu I learned that we are born as vessels open to the life force (*prana*), which I understand also as the Holy Spirit—that life force that animates us and all creatures. As we move from infancy through childhood to adulthood, our minds become "overgrown," cutting us off from the wisdom of the heart and body. In the Episcopal Church we identify closely with the Enlightenment virtue of rational thought, of question-wrestling and reasoning. Scientists and intellectuals find a home in the Episcopal Church in a way they don't in other, more dogmatic denominations. But unchecked, our strength can become our weakness, and our minds can become dense and impenetrable thickets that prevent the heart and bodily expressions of our humanity. We "Frozen Chosen" need to guard against that especially.

Yogic philosophy offers an alternative to either-or thinking about the body and spirit, for in yoga the body becomes the very key that unlocks the door to the spirit, to kingdom living, to the peace of God. When Jesus said, "The Kingdom of Heaven is within you" (Luke 17:21, NKJV), he meant the kingdom is within our mortal, human bodies. God considers our bodies—imperfect, frail, flawed, and unreliable as they may be—suitable and fit containers to hold paradise. This body is where we meet God, and a high regard for the human body is necessary if we are to imagine these vessels as meeting places for the Divine.

---

48. *The Book of Common Prayer*, 491.

49. Paul, *Jesus in the Lotus*, 27–29.

50. Paul, *Jesus in the Lotus*, 30.

3

THEOLOGICAL ENCOUNTERS AT THE APEX

> Let the beauty we love be what we do.
> There are hundreds of ways to kneel and kiss the ground.[1]
>
> –*Rumi*

> As a tethered bird grows tired of flying about in vain to find a place of rest and settles down at last on its own perch, so the mind, tired of wandering about hither and thither, settles down at last in the Self, dear one, to which it is bound. All creatures, dear one, have their source in him. He is their home; he is their strength.
>
> –*The Chandogya Upanishad, 6.8*[2]

> [O Lord], You move us to delight in praising You; for You have made us for Yourself, and our hearts are restless until they find rest in You.
>
> –*St. Augustine,* Confessions, *Book 1.1*

READ YOGIC PHILOSOPHY and you will begin to discover many parallels between it and Christian Holy Scripture. Texts such as the Upanishads, the Bhagavad Gita, or the Yoga Sutras of Patanjali brim with teachings that send the curious in search of places in the Bible where Jesus or Paul said much the same thing. This is hardly surprising, for the ancient world was crisscrossed by trade routes, facilitating the exchange of not only goods but ideas. Cynthia Bourgeault cautions us against sentimentalizing Jesus as an uneducated carpenter's son from a dusty village of no consequence who learned everything he needed to know directly from God.[3]

Pointing to the tendency to see Jerusalem as the cultural center of the ancient world, Bourgeault says that "Galilee was actually the more cosmopolitan environment because it lay on the Silk Road, that great viaduct of human

1. Coleman Barks, *Rumi: The Big Red Book: The Great Masterpiece Celebrating Mystical Love and Friendship* (New York: HarperOne, 2011), 367.

2. Upanishads, 133–34.

3. Bourgeault, *The Wisdom Jesus*, 25.

commerce which from time immemorial has connected the lands of the Mediterranean with the lands and culture of Central Asia and China. The Silk Road went right through Capernaum, where Jesus did a lot of his learning and teaching."[4] The bustling and wealthy city of Sepphoris was an easy walk from Nazareth, and its marketplace offered an array of both domestic and foreign goods. In other words, the teachings and ministry of Jesus did not evolve in a cultural vacuum.

That religions shape one another is not news. Any student of Christianity learns that the teachings of Jesus were presented through different lenses according to the evangelist reporting them: Matthew presented through the lens of Judaism, and John through a more Hellenistic lens.

So, if one examines the wisdom tradition running beneath yogic philosophy and Christianity, many theological parallels can be seen. The goal is not to collapse two great religious and philosophical traditions into one, but rather to delight at the places where they teach their adherents the same things. We can even gain new insight into Christian scriptures by looking at them through the lens of Eastern philosophy, especially when we read some of the mystical or more puzzling teachings of Jesus.

In this chapter, I offer a look at some of those parallels, drawing on Pantanjali's Yoga Sutras and on Eknath Easwaran's translations of the Upanishads and the Bhagavad Gita. Easwaran was born, educated, and taught college in India. He came to the United States in 1959 as a Fulbright Scholar and stayed on to teach and write. He became a prolific author, a researcher, and an authority on spiritual practice. His translations are accessible and beautifully introduced.

Each of the following sections represents a theological parallel I have encountered between yogic and Christian texts, and I suspect I have only begun to till the ground where many more lie slumbering. Once you find a parallel, others seem to attach themselves to it, and before you know it you have an entire meditation. Any one of the following meeting places between yogic philosophy and Christian scripture would be an excellent foundation for a Yoga in the Church workshop. Undoubtedly, as you read, pray, and study you will find many more.

Love Your Neighbor as Yourself—See God in All

Compassionate, expansive regard or *agape* love for the other is the kind of love God has for us. It is a concept important in both yogic philosophy and

4. Bourgeault, *The Wisdom Jesus*, 25.

Christianity. In the following passages, the implication is that such love identifies one as a disciple (or one seeking enlightenment), and in the New Testament, discipleship is the highest state of spiritual union available in this mortal life. Spiritual union with God is another way of expressing the concept of eternal life.

> When a person responds to the joys and sorrows of others as if they were his own, he has attained the highest state of spiritual union. (Bhagavad Gita 6:32)
>
> But those who worship me with love live in me, and I come to life in them. (Bhagavad Gita 9:29)
>
> By this everyone will know that you are my disciples, if you have love for one another. (John 13:35)
>
> "Teacher, which commandment in the law is the greatest?" He said to him, "'You shall love the Lord your God with all your heart, and with all your soul, and with all your mind.' This is the greatest and first commandment. And a second is like it: 'You shall love your neighbor as yourself.' On these two commandments hang all the law and the prophets." (Matt. 22:36–40)
>
> For you were called to freedom, brothers and sisters; only do not use your freedom as an opportunity for self-indulgence, but through love become slaves to one another. For the whole law is summed up in a single commandment, "You shall love your neighbor as yourself." (Gal. 5:13–14)
>
> You shall love your neighbor as yourself . . . (Lev. 19:18)

In Pali, a liturgical language of North India, the word *metta* describes the principal of lovingkindness. It is a foundational virtue recognized by Buddhism as a heavenly or divine abode.[5] Lovingkindness is the dwelling place of the divine. Metta and agape have much in common. If we regard Jesus's teaching to love one another *only* as a golden rule for helping us get along with folks, *only* as a means to ensure society behaves itself, then we tragically miss the invitation into the divine abode. Consider instead that Jesus's teaching is showing us the doorway into participation in the divine life. If you love one another, if you love your neighbor as yourself, then—when you do that—you will be dwelling with God. You will be participating—in real time—in the life of God.

Buddhist meditation teacher Sharon Salzberg explains that the word *metta* "has two root meanings. One is the word for 'gentle.' Metta is likened to a gentle

5. Sharon Salzberg, *Lovingkindness: The Revolutionary Art of Happiness* (Boulder, CO: Shambala Publications, 2002), 18.

rain that falls upon the earth. This rain does not select or choose . . . it simply falls without discrimination."[6] The other root meaning is "friend"—the kind of friend who is a constant refuge, a helper and protector, one who "will not forsake us when we are in trouble nor rejoice in our misfortune."[7] This "friend" aspect of metta sounds very similar to the language of psalms used to describe God:

> God is our refuge and strength, a very present help in trouble. (Ps. 46:1)
>
> God is my helper; the Lord is the upholder of my life. (Ps. 54:4)
>
> [The Lord is] my rock and my fortress, my stronghold and my deliverer, my shield, in whom I take refuge. (Ps. 144:2)

In the fifth chapter (verses 43–45) of Matthew's Gospel, Jesus speaks of loving one's neighbor (including one's enemy) and says that the Father in heaven sends rain on the righteous and unrighteous alike:

> "You have heard that it was said, 'You shall love your neighbor and hate your enemy.' But I say to you, Love your enemies and pray for those who persecute you, so that you may be children of your Father in heaven; for he makes his sun rise on the evil and on the good, and sends rain on the righteous and on the unrighteous."

If read narrowly, this passage reeks of unfairness. What is the point of our good behavior if God is going to reward the bad guys in equal measure to us? If, however, you read this passage more expansively, it says that because God is metta—because the divine nature is lovingkindness—it is the nature of God to love without discrimination. God simply cannot help being God.

Be One as the Father and I Are One–You Are That

Eknath Easwaran turns to one of the Upanishadic texts—the Chandogya Upanishad, dating from around 600 BCE—to explain the relationship between the individual and the absolute. God immanent (God within us) is called *Atman*, and God transcendent is called *Brahman*. Easwaran writes, "In the climax of

6. Salzberg, *Lovingkindness*, 24.
7. Salzberg, *Lovingkindness*, 24.

meditation, the sages discovered unity: the same indivisible reality without and within."[8] Atman *is* Brahman.

> Tat tvam asi, or Thou art That. This is also expressed as You are That! [This line repeats throughout the chapter.] (Chandogya Upanishad, 6.2.3)
>
> [Jesus said,] "I ask not only on behalf of these, but also on behalf of those who will believe in me through their word, that they may all be one. As you, Father, are in me and I am in you, may they also be in us, so that the world may believe that you have sent me. The glory that you have given me I have given them, so that they may be one, as we are one, I in them and you in me, that they may become completely one, so that the world may know that you have sent me and have loved them even as you have loved me. (John 17:20–23)

It is the God immanent, the God within, the image of God in every single one of us that unites us each personally with God and unites us communally with one another. Galatians 3:28 points to this inner unifying presence or image: "There is no longer Jew or Greek, there is no longer slave or free, there is no longer male and female; for all of you are one in Christ Jesus."

Easwaran explains that the Upanishads teach

> there is a Reality underlying life which rituals cannot reach, next to which the things we see and touch in everyday life are shadows. . . . [T]his Reality is the essence of every created thing, and the same Reality is our real Self, so that each of us is one with the power that created and sustains the universe. And, finally, they teach that this oneness can be realized directly, without the mediation of priests or rituals or any of the structures of organized religion, not after death but in this life, and that this is the purpose for which each of us has been born and the goal toward which evolution moves.[9]

What Easwaran calls "Reality" I understand as God transcendent, and what he calls "Self," God immanent or God within. When these expressions of the divine are in sync, in union, both in an individual and in societies, then creation begins to manifest what the Jewish tradition calls *shalom* and Pierre Teilhard de Chardin called the *Omega Point*. The Bible is bookended by depictions of this manifestation: in Genesis, in the Garden before the Fall, and at the

8. Bhagavad Gita, 26.
9. Upanishads, 22.

end in the Revelation of John, in the harmonious and fruitful "New Jerusalem." This shalom is both our origin and the home toward which we travel.

Nonduality

Just as there is a unity or oneness between the God within us and the God without—the God transcendent—it follows that there is a unity or oneness between the person and the world. A nondualist, a unitive thinker, does not regard the world first and foremost in terms of distinctions or opposites, does not see the world primarily as a system of categories or divisions (useful as the science of taxonomy may be), does not live in a state of us-and-them thinking. Jesus's "love your neighbor as yourself" teachings are basically about trying to get us to view the world as more unitive thinkers. The mind of Christ was a unitive, nondual mind. There is an inherent irony in using a counterpoint of yogic and Christian scriptures to compare what each says about unity.

In Colossians 3:1–11, Paul explains that if one has been raised with Christ, one should be seeking things that are "above" earthly concerns. This means the "putting to death" of "whatever in you is earthly: fornication, impurity, passion, evil desire, and greed." These actions all arise from dualistic thinking, from regarding the other as an object instead of as akin to and in some respects indistinguishable from oneself. Paul describes these as the practices of "the old self"—the dualistic thinking self—and reminds the Colossians they have "clothed [themselves] with the new self, which is being renewed in knowledge according to the image of its creator." The "new self" is the nondualist, the unitive thinker who sees as does Christ. To underscore the "death" of divisions, categories, and labels in the new self, Paul concludes, "In that renewal there is no longer Greek and Jew, circumcised and uncircumcised, barbarian, Scythian, slave and free; but Christ is all and in all!"

The Brihadaranyaka Upanishad (dating from around 700 BCE) 4.22 also speaks of the meaninglessness of divisions and their irrelevance to the Self—the God within: "In that unitive state there is neither father nor mother, neither worlds nor gods nor even scriptures. In that state there is neither thief nor slayer, neither low caste nor high, neither monk nor ascetic. The Self is beyond good and evil, beyond all suffering of the human heart."[10] In yogic thought, the lowercase "self" means "ego," and "Self" with a capital S means the God within or the Atman.

10. Upanishads, 111.

A division or distinction that gets a great deal of attention in the New Testament is that of Jew and Gentile. In Ephesians 2:11–22, Paul assures his audience that Jesus Christ has reconciled Jews and Gentiles and that they are one in him. Verses 13 through 16 speak of Christ "creat[ing] in himself one new humanity in place of the two, thus making peace, and [reconciling] both groups to God in one body through the cross, thus putting to death that hostility through it." In Christ, the hostility borne of dualistic us-versus-them thinking has been put to death by love.

Russill Paul observes that Jesus used parables to "help people who are stuck in the details of religion to move into the spirit of it, or in Eastern terms, to move from dualistic to non-dualistic consciousness."[11] In at least two parables (the prodigal son and the laborers in the vineyard) the theme of fairness and unfairness presents the kingdom of heaven as nondualistic and invites the listener to move there from a dualistic perspective.

The mind of God, the mind of Jesus Christ, is a unitive, nondualistic mind, a mind that values participation over competition, a mind that sees wholeness instead of division. We come into the world as unitive thinkers. As infants we naturally inhabit the mind of Christ. When we learn to walk, we must be taught to be dualistic, binary thinkers to ensure our own survival. For example, if we are not taught to discern between the safety of a parent versus the potential risk of a stranger, or the safety of a sidewalk versus the potential danger of a street, or the safety of a tabletop versus the potential danger of a hot stove, we might not survive childhood. Some measure of dualistic or binary thinking is essential for survival. But we can get stuck there, convinced it's the only way or the right way to see the world. The Christian journey can be thought of as the journey from dualistic or binary thinking back to nondualistic or unitive thinking. I think this is what Jesus means in Matthew 18:3 when he says, "Unless you change and become like little children, you will never enter the kingdom of heaven." Unless you stop dividing the world into them and us, you'll never find union with God.

In John 3:3–7 Jesus calls this change into unitive thinking being "born from above." The Jewish Pharisee Nicodemus interprets Jesus's words literally and is mightily confused about how he's supposed to manage re-entering his mother's womb to be born again. Jesus clarifies that it is a birth "of water and Spirit" that gains one entry into—allows one "to see"—the kingdom of God. I offer this to underscore an important distinction between yogic philosophy and Christianity:

11. Paul, *Jesus in the Lotus,* 101.

In the former, it is the practitioner who strives toward union with God. In the latter, it is a gift from God (that gift is "Spirit"), presumably together with the believer's choice to be baptized ("water"), that constitutes a *mutual* striving—a mutual reaching forth of God to humanity and humanity to God.

The Katha Upanishad (dating from around 500–800 BCE) 2.3.10–11 teaches that "when the five senses are stilled, when the mind is stilled, when the intellect is stilled, that is called the highest state by the wise. They say yoga is this complete stillness in which one enters the unitive state."[12] Here is another seeming distinction: the Upanishad teaches stillness as a way to enter the unitive state, and Jesus teaches love as a way to enter it. Perhaps we need not choose between the two approaches. Perhaps, it is simply from interior stillness, from a unitive state, that agape love or metta best arise and flourish.

Recall that yoga is a practice of seeking union with God, with Brahman, with the divine by whatever name. So, stilling the body, mind, and senses is a yoga. Practicing love is a yoga. (If yoga is understood in this way, then to some degree all the sacraments could be seen as a yoga, for in all of them we seek union with God, and to be oriented toward union is to begin to see as a nondualist.) Jesus taught his friends about love as a way of not only harmonizing and gentling the world, but as a way of finding union with God—a way of living in nonduality.

In Luke 11:34 Jesus says, "Your eye is the lamp of your body. If your eye is healthy, your whole body is full of light; but if it is not healthy, your body is full of darkness." The Greek απλουσ [*haplous*], often translated "healthy," can also mean "single" (as in single-visioned), "single-minded," or "unitive."[13] When we see the world with single-mindedness—with the unitive mind—we will be filled with the light of Christ. The footnotes to this verse in the NIV translation (which also renders it "healthy") state that the Greek word implies generosity. To see with generosity is to engage the unitive mind.

That opens new meaning in the post-Communion prayer, when we often say: "Send us now into the world in peace, and grant us strength and courage to love and serve you with gladness and singleness of heart."[14] God, may we serve you with gladness, with a unitive heart and mind, and with a generosity of seeing. This is the last prayer we say together on Sunday morning, as we seek to strengthen the faltering ability most of us have in living faithfully in the world.

---

12. Upanishads, 91.

13. James Strong, *The Exhaustive Concordance of the Bible* (Cincinnati: Jennings & Graham, 1890), No. 573. Hereafter referred to as Strong's Greek Concordance.

14. *The Book of Common Prayer*, 365.

It is devilishly hard to live to live in the world in nonduality. As one of my favorite seminary professors—a character who minced no words and delighted in shocking us seminarians out of our classroom torpor—used to say, "I leave church on Sunday and I'm doing a great job of loving my neighbor, until some sonofabitch cuts me off in traffic." For most of us, our capacity to actually live in nonduality is fleeting and tenuous at best. Thankfully, spiritual practices such as yoga teach us to gradually stretch those fleeting moments into more sustained ways of being.

Putting the Ego in Its Place

There's nothing wrong with having an ego. An ego is part of the package we come with. The peril is in mistaking the ego for the Self. The very genesis of sin in the Bible is when people confuse the two, putting themselves (their "selfs" or egos) in the place of God.

As Episcopalian Christians with a high anthropology (a high regard for the human person in all its gorgeous expressions of diversity), the ego is part of what it means to be human and part of how our diversity gets expressed. To cast away the ego would in some sense be dishonoring our humanity and our diversity. Let us agree, then, that the ego has its place—a place subordinate to the Self, subordinate to the God or the Christ within. The work is to keep the ego in its place, to keep things in the correct order. We invite trouble when we greet the world through the ego alone or when we try to love through the ego alone.

How do we subordinate the ego to the Christ within? Yogic philosophy and Christianity seem to agree that the way is through renunciation of attachment to things other than God. If you associate the word *renunciation* with "monastic" and "vows of poverty," and think, *Whoa, not me*, you're not alone. But maybe renunciation needn't be all or nothing. Perhaps the practice of moderation (in Sanskrit, *brahmacarya*) offers training wheels for those of us for whom renunciation seems too unattainable and severe.

In his introduction to the Bhagavad Gita, Easwaran says that although *renunciation* is a bleak word in English, it is the very essence of the Bhagavad Gita. The text promises freedom through renunciation, and yet

> the impression most of us get is that we are being asked to give up everything we want out of life; in this drab state, having lost whatever we value, we will be free from sorrow. Who wants that kind of freedom?

> But this is not at all what the Gita means. It does not even enjoin material renunciation, although it certainly encourages simplicity. As always, its emphasis is on the mind. It teaches that we can become free by giving up not material things, but selfish attachments to material things—and, more important, to people. It asks us to renounce not the enjoyment of life, but the clinging to selfish enjoyment whatever it may cost others. It pleads, in a word, for the renunciation of selfishness in thought, word, and action—a theme that is common to all mystics, West and East alike.[15]

Although not necessarily coequal with yogic philosophy, Tibetan Buddhism, according to meditation teacher Sharon Salzberg, "defines renunciation as accepting what comes into our lives and letting go of what leaves our lives. To renounce in this sense is to come to a state of simple being."[16] Christian contemplative James Finley echoes this in his statement that "a simple openness to the next human moment brings us into union with God in Christ."[17] Renunciation can be a far more gentle and gradual process than we might at first imagine upon encountering the word.

In the canon of Christian scripture, other writers say the same thing, that if we allow the transient attractions and cares of the world to consume our desire and attention, we will be unable to manifest the love of the Father—agape love, or metta. Consider the first letter of John and the letter to the Colossians:

> Do not love the world or the things in the world. If anyone loves the world, the love of the Father is not in him. For all that is in the world—the desires of the flesh and the desires of the eyes and pride in possessions—is not from the Father but is from the world. And the world is passing away along with its desires, but whoever does the will of God abides forever. (1 John 2:15–17 ESV)

> Set your minds on things that are above, not on things that are on earth. (Col. 3:2)

The letter of James states this more strongly, depicting those of us who cling to the world as the actual adversaries of God: "You adulterous people! Do you not know that friendship with the world is enmity with God? Therefore, whoever wishes to be a friend of the world makes himself an enemy of God" (4:4 ESV).

15. Bhagavad Gita, 51.

16. Salzberg, *Lovingkindness*, 55.

17. The Rt. Rev. Frank Grisworld, homily, Episcopal Diocese of Chicago, Diocesan Convention, February 26, 1994.

In the twelfth chapter of the Bhagavad Gita, Krishna—the god of tenderness, love, and compassion—expresses the same sentiment in the positive, saying that he loves those who live "beyond the reach of 'I' and 'mine,'" those who are "not agitating the world or agitated by it [and who] stand above the sway of elation, competition, and fear."[18] In other words, it would appear that James and Krishna agree that people who are totally self-focused and consumed by the fleeting and moment-to-moment dramas of worldly life are completely missing the mark.

Putting our ego in its place is something that Christian prayer and service as well as the practice of yoga all support. Salzberg says that the ability to get out of our self-centeredness is not a matter of it being a skill some of us are born with and others not. Rather, she says, it's the result "of what we do with our minds: We can choose to transform our minds so that they embody love, or we can allow them to develop habits and false concepts of separation."[19]

Paul, in Romans 12:2 ESV, also advocates standing apart from the world and looking to the mind to open oneself to the process of transformation. In brackets I have included alternate meanings for some of the Greek: "Do not be conformed to [don't assimilate into, or fashion yourself after, or be formed by] this world, but be [spiritually] transformed by the renewal of your [intellect] mind, that by testing you may discern what is the will [pleasure, purpose] of God, what is good [generous] and acceptable [well-pleasing] and perfect [fully developed, complete]."

Cynthia Bourgeault feels that in many of his teachings, Jesus's principal target is not religious authorities or empires, but the egoic mind: "[Jesus] is very deliberately trying to short-circuit that grasping, acquiring, clinging, comparing linear brain and to open up within us a whole new mode of perception (not what we see, but *how* we see; how the mind makes its connections)."[20] Elsewhere, Bourgeault calls this "the large mind" and says that going into the large mind is a valid translation of *metanoia*, to repent. [21] Jesus's call to repent because the kingdom of heaven is at hand is thus not only a call to be sincerely remorseful for our sins and offenses and to humbly ask for Christ's help to do better, it also stands as a call to go into the large mind—to go to the way of seeing and thinking that puts our ego in its place, subordinate to the God within

18. Bhagavad Gita, 208–9.

19. Salzberg, *Lovingkindness*, 89.

20. Bourgeault, *The Wisdom Jesus*, 50–51.

21. Bourgeault, *The Wisdom Jesus*, 37.

us. This is where transformation happens. This is where we can begin to escape entrapment in the endless cycle of sin and repentance. This is where we can fully receive the forgiveness that is offered us in Christ.

Understanding the subordination of the ego as the subordination of the self to the Self opens up interesting possibilities for interpreting several Christian scriptures. In John 3:30 (NIV), John the Baptist says of Jesus, "He must become greater; I must become less." Considering this metaphorically, what if John the Baptist stands for the self and Jesus for the Self; John the Baptist represents the ego and Jesus the unitive or "large" mind? And in Luke 22:42, when Jesus speaks that deeply human line from the Garden of Gethsemane—"Father, if you are willing, remove this cup from me; yet, not my will but yours be done"—perhaps he is giving us a glimpse into this process at work—the process of subordinating the human ego to the mind of God.

"Let the same mind be in you that was in Christ Jesus," wrote Paul to the Philippians (2:5)—large, unitive, grasping at and clinging to nothing, fully at home in the will of God.

Abiding in God

Both the Bhagavad Gita and Christian scripture say something about the inseparability of God and humanity. We are bound together, we and God. When we realize that and live accordingly, we bear fruit, and we enjoy the presence of God.

In the Gita (6:30–31), Krishna says, "I am ever present to those who have realized me in every creature. Seeing all life as my manifestation, they are never separated from me. They worship me in the hearts of all. And all their actions proceed from me. Wherever they live, they abide in me."

In the Gospel of John, Jesus says, "Abide in me as I abide in you. Just as the branch cannot bear fruit by itself unless it abides in the vine, neither can you unless you abide in me" (15:4).

In the extracanonical *Gospel of Thomas*, saying 77 echoes the Bhagavad Gita's assertion that all life manifests the divine: Jesus said, "It is I who am the light (that presides) over all. It is I who am the entirety: it is from me that the entirety has come, and to me that the entirety goes. Split a piece of wood: I am there. Lift a stone, and you [plural] will find me there."[22]

---

22. "Gospel of Thomas Commentary," Gospel of Thomas Commentary, accessed October 18, 2021, *http://www.earlychristianwritings.com/thomas/*.

Finding the divine *in* the world holds in check the temptation to turn away from or reject the world in order to find God. For all their focus on stilling and withdrawing from the chatter of life, both the Bhagavad Gita and Christian scripture are ultimately concerned with how to live *in the world* as a person in sync with God. Otherwise, their relevance for us would be thin.

It's Not Easy to Enter the Kingdom of Heaven or to Attain Supreme Consciousness

I will confess I've always resented Jesus for urging us to repent because the kingdom of heaven is at hand but then adding elsewhere that it'll be hard to enter that kingdom and that not everyone will make it. Inviting us forward and then holding us at arm's length always felt confusing and rather mean-spirited to me, even as I knew such an interpretation was off-base because it was incompatible with the nature of God.

I think Peter would agree with me: after he hears Jesus tell the parable of the rich young man (Matthew 19:16–26; the disciples' reaction is also found in Luke 18:24–27), Peter expresses the exasperation of the disciples when he says to Jesus, "Look we've left everything to follow you, and now you're telling us that may not even be sufficient?" Jesus has just warned his disciples that "it is easier for a camel to go through the eye of a needle than for someone who is rich to enter the kingdom of God," and the disciples' reaction is typically translated as "greatly astounded" or "greatly amazed." The Greek words can also mean "to violently strike someone out of their wits."[23] In other words, Jesus has just smacked the disciples upside the head with his words, meaning that those words must point to a critically important teaching. Jesus concludes by inferring that salvation (or having eternal life) is impossible for mortals alone and requires the action of God.

Mortals can't do this, but God can. With God all things are possible. Because God is compassionate and overflowing with grace, it will be possible to enter the kingdom. That puts us in the tenuous position of trying hard and then waiting around for God to decide to admit us. But what if we read this story with the knowledge of the self and the Self—the ego and the Atman, or God within? We clinging, grasping, materially focused egoic mortals can't enter union with God, but through the ego-less Self (the God within, or the Atman) and *by the grace of God transcendent* (not the God within but the God *without*, the Brahman) we are actually able to enter the kingdom. The sliver of

23. Strong's Greek Concordance, Nos. 4970, 4141, 1605.

God within us (so slim Jesus calls it the eye of a needle) serves as the portal into divine life. It isn't easy, but it is possible. Reading the parable this way gives us not control but at least a little agency. Without the lush grace of God, we can go nowhere, but at least we can really believe we might be able to step inside when Jesus tells us the kingdom is near.

The Katha Upanishad 1.3.14 uses the image of a razor to describe the difficulty of the path that leads to union with God: "Get up! Wake up! Seek the guidance of an illumined teacher and realize the Self. Sharp like a razor's edge, the sages say, is the path, difficult to traverse."[24] Swami Mukundananda, reflecting on the words of the fifteenth-century Indian mystic and poet Kabir Das, likewise describes the path of love as narrow—too narrow to accommodate the ego: "When 'I' existed, God was not there; now God exists and 'I' do not. The path of divine love is very narrow; it cannot accommodate both 'I' and God."[25]

A razor-sharp path, an impossibly small needle eye, a narrow gate, and a hard road—both Eastern and Western scriptures are frank about how hard it is to enter the kingdom and find union with God. What if we are tiny (but marvelous) bits of the essence of God wrapped in countless layers of human flesh and will? As Hindu Roman Catholic Raimon Panikkar puts it, there is a "deep inner center in the human person with the capacity to manifest Christ."[26] If we insist on bringing our lumbering egos along, they make it impossible for us to push our way through the narrow gate by means of force. The art is to enter instead through the tiny and marvelous God bit within us, the "deep inner center"—a kernel that, sadly, many of us don't even know we possess.

Dharma, Ahimsa, Physics, and What You Do to the Least

The concepts of *dharma* and *karma* are foundational to the Bhagavad Gita. I think of dharma as a principle of stillness and solidness, and karma as one of movement or action of the body or the thoughts. Easwaran explains that the root of the word *dharma* means "to support, to hold up or bear." He says that "generally dharma implies support from within: the essence of a thing, its

24. Upanishads, 82.

25. "Bhagavad Gita: Chapter 13, Verse 8–12," Bhagavad Gita: The Song of God, accessed October 18, 2021, *https://www.holy-bhagavad-gita.org/chapter/13/verse/8–12.*

See also V.V. Subba Rao, *The Bhagavad Gita Sri Krishna Arjuna Samvaada: A Study* (Morrisville, NC: Lulu, 2019), 121.

26. Ilia Delio, *Christ in Evolution* (Maryknoll, NY: Orbis Books, 2008), 89, quoting Panikkar, "A Christophany for Our Time," *Theology Digest* 39, no.1 (Spring 1992): 3–21.

virtue, that which makes it what it is."[27] Dharma is the collection of beams and two-by-fours that hold up a house, or the collection of bones and sinews that hold up the bodies in which we each live. You don't mess with dharma without inviting chaos. Try to open and close a door after a large tree falls on your roof and smashes a wall. Try walking with a broken femur.

Because dharma is so essential to "integrity and harmony in the universe," it means by extension that which is right, good, and just. Because all things in creation are linked together, a disruption of dharma over here means some impact will be felt over there. Easwaran notes that the sages of the Upanishads discovered "that all things are interconnected because at its deepest level creation is indivisible."[28] Recent discoveries in quantum mechanics affirm this.

Quantum physicists theorize that beneath the molecular level of electrons, quarks, and neutrinos, all matter is comprised of quivering strings. Everything—from the chair you are sitting on to the lungs you are breathing with—is comprised of these strings. Different kinds of matter have different vibrational patterns and frequencies. In other words, the superstrings in your chair vibrate at a different frequency and pattern than do the ones in your lungs. The frequency or pattern of the vibration of the superstrings determines the nature of the matter they manifest. What a great hiding place for God this would be: at the ultramicroscopic level of matter!

Maybe the psalmist had the mind of a physicist when he said to God, "Where can I go from your Spirit? Where can I flee from your presence? If I go up to the heavens you are there; If I make my bed in the depths, you are there" (139:7–8 NIV). If God is in fact present, in the heavens and the underworld and everywhere in between, dancing among the strings at the submolecular level, it also opens new possibilities for understanding the parable of the sheep and goats, especially the takeaway line, "Just as you did it to one of the least of these who are members of my family, you did it to me" (Matt. 25:40b).

The Greek that is usually translated "did" can also mean "caused an effect." The Greek that is usually translated "least" can also mean "smallest in size." The Greek for "member of my family" may also be translated "brother," or literally, "one of the same womb."[29]

27. Bhagavad Gita, 31.

28. Bhagavad Gita, 32.

29. (1) epoihsate from poiew [Strong's #4160] has many meanings, among them, "you caused an effect, you treated, you brought evil on or inflicted"; (2) Strong's #1646, elacistos superlative of mikros [Strong's #3398] means "little, small in size, quantity," etc. (3) Brother or "someone from the same womb" adelfwn from adelfos [Strong's #80] is related to delfus "womb," a word from which comes "dolphin," a fish with a womb. Interestingly, the dolphin was a prominent symbol in early Christian art, one rich with meaning.

Richard Rohr reflects on the visions of the fourteenth-century mystic Julian of Norwich and declares that we "come from the Womb of the Eternal. We are not simply made by God; we are made 'of God.'" He writes that according to Julian, God is in the very substance of creation and can be smelled, tasted, and swallowed.[30]

Whatever you do to one of the least of these who are members of my family, you do to me. We can hear these words from two voices, both of them valid and valuable to our faith. If we hear Jesus speak these words, then the least are those on the margins of society—the poor and vulnerable he is always reminding us to consider. If we hear these words being spoken by the cosmic and eternal Christ, then the meaning of the least or the smallest can rightly expand to include all matter. This is a Christ-centered view of the cosmos instead of a human-centered one. The body of Christ encompasses the cosmos—a view that theologians from Raimon Panikkar to Pierre Teilhard de Chardin to Ilia Delio share in common—and "member of my family" can mean a blade of grass, a redwood, a hawk, the fragment of a star, or a single-celled organism, as well as the molecules that comprise them. The discovery of the Upanishads thus stands: that at its deepest level creation is indivisible, and all things are interconnected. There is nothing in creation that does not share kinship with the Christ.

"I am ever present to those who have realized me in every creature," says the Bhagavad Gita (6:30–32). "Seeing all life as my manifestation, they are never separated from me. They worship me in the hearts of all, and all their actions proceed from me. Wherever they may live, they abide in me."[31]

Our treatment of the divine in all creation is governed by *ahimsa*, the Sanskrit word for nonviolence, for universal love for all creatures. To violate the principle of ahimsa—to do violence to another—is to threaten the very integrity of dharma, to take an ax to the beams that uphold the house. This is expressed by the ancient epigram *ahimsa paramo dharma*: "There is no higher dharma than nonviolence."[32]

This leads us to karma—and to mustard seeds.

---

30. Richard Rohr, "Our Deepest Desire," Center for Action and Contemplation," May 30, 2019, *https://cac.org/our-deepest-desire-2019-05-30/*.

31. Bhagavad Gita, 143.

32. Upanishads, 326.

Karma, Reaping and Sowing, and Mustard Seeds

The law of karma states that every action has a consequence, and every consequence in turn has consequences. Whatever we do ripples outward from us, touching other beings in ways we often do not and will never know. These ripples extend outward from every being that has agency, forming a web of interconnectedness comprised of cause and effect—a web of the activity of life.

Easwaran explains that karma

> refers not only to physical action but to mental activity as well. In their analysis of the phenomenal world and the world within, the sages of the Upanishads found that there is not merely an accidental but an essential relationship between mental and physical activity. Given appropriate conditions to develop further, thoughts breed actions of the same kind, as a seed can grow only into one particular kind of tree.[33]

You can sense something of the law of karma at work in Paul's letters to the Galatians (6:7–8) and the Corinthians (2 Cor. 9:6). In Galatians, Paul writes, "Do not be deceived; God is not mocked, for you reap whatever you sow. If you sow to your own flesh, you will reap corruption from the flesh; but if you sow to the Spirit, you will reap eternal life from the Spirit." What goes around comes around, and God is not mocked—literally: do not wrinkle up your nose in derision or contempt for God.[34] In Eastern words, you cannot outsmart the law of karma, which was given to us to guide us toward enduring truth, toward dharma.

In the sixth chapter of the Gospel of Luke (vv. 27–38), Jesus teaches about loving one's enemies and giving of one's goods without condition. "Do to others as you would have them do to you," he says, suggesting a karmic connection between the actions of two people. "Do not judge, and you will not be judged; do not condemn, and you will not be condemned. Forgive, and you will be forgiven; give, and it will be given to you. A good measure, pressed down, shaken together, running over, will be put into your lap; for the measure you give will be the measure you get back."

Easwaran notes, "The law of karma states unequivocally that though we cannot see the connections, we can be sure that everything that happens to us, good and bad, originated once in something we did or thought. . . . [It] is in

---

33. Bhagavad Gita, 33.

34. Strong's Greek Concordance, No. 3456.

the mind rather than the world that karma's seeds are planted."[35] A tiny seed of a thought, he says, can take root opportunistically and grow and spread into something beyond our control. Yoga can help tame the mind so that seeds are planted not recklessly but with intention, and so yoga becomes a valuable discipline as we work to undo patterns of negative thinking.

This calls to mind the parable of the mustard seed (Matt. 13:31–32): "[Jesus] put before them another parable: 'The kingdom of heaven is like a mustard seed that someone took and sowed in his field; it is the smallest of all the seeds, but when it has grown it is the greatest of shrubs and becomes a tree, so that the birds of the air come and make nests in its branches.'" If the kingdom of heaven is within us (Luke 17:21), then a tiny seed of a thought has the power to plant something that grows vigorously, far beyond anything we might imagine when it is planted. What is produced from that seed is either negative and destructive or positive and beneficial to others beyond ourselves. It is ours to choose.

I Am Beginning, Middle, End–the Alpha and the Omega

Alpha A and omega Ω—the first and last letters of the Greek alphabet—were a staple of early Christian art on the walls of catacombs, tile mosaic floors, stone carvings, and painted icons. From the beginning, the paired letters have been used to express the infinitude and eternal nature of God.[36]

Considered by some to be one of the earliest Christian mystics,[37] Clement of Alexandria (ca. 150–215 CE) wrote of Jesus, "He is the circle of all powers rolled and united into one unity. For that reason, the Word [Jesus] is called the Alpha and the Omega, of whom alone the end becomes the beginning. . . . For that reason, also, to believe in Him and by Him, is to become a unity, being indissolubly united in Him."[38]

In the Revelation of John (22:13), Jesus referred to himself as eternal: "I am the Alpha and the Omega, the first and the last, the beginning and the end." He also stated this in Revelation 1:8 and 21:6. In making this claim, Jesus is declaring himself to be the eternal Christ. As Richard Rohr puts it,

35. Bhagavad Gita, 34.

36. F. L. Cross and E. A. Livingstone, eds., *The Oxford Dictionary of the Christian Church* (Oxford: Oxford University Press, 1997), 45.

37. Carl McColman, *The Big Book of Christian Mysticism: The Essential Guide to Contemplative Spirituality* (Charlottesville, VA: Hampton Roads Publishing, 2010), 48.

38. David W. Bercot, ed., *A Dictionary of Early Christian Beliefs* (Peabody, MA: Hendrickson Publishers, 1998), 370.

> Christ is eternal; Jesus was born in time. Jesus without Christ invariably becomes time and culturally bound, which excludes much of humanity from Christ's embrace. Christ without Jesus easily becomes an abstract metaphysics or a mere ideology without personal engagement or passion. Love always needs a direct object. We need them both and thus we rightly believe in both, Jesus and Christ, just as most Christians would verbally say.[39]

The Bhagavad Gita likewise speaks of the infinitude and eternal nature of God. Krishna says, "I am the true Self in the heart of every creature . . . and the beginning, middle, and end of their existence."[40] He also says, "Among words, [I am] the syllable Om[41]; among purifying forces, I am the wind";[42] "I am the beginning, middle, and end of creation"; [43] "I am the seed that can be found in every creature . . . for without me nothing can exist, neither animate nor inanimate."[44] "Just remember that I am, and that I support the entire cosmos with only a fragment of my being."[45]

God supports the entire cosmos with only a fragment of the divine being. Consider this alongside Psalm 8, wherein the psalmist describes the heavens as the work of God's fingers:

> When I look at your heavens, the work of your fingers,
> the moon and the stars that you have established;
> what are human beings that you are mindful of them,
> mortals that you care for them? (vv. 3–4)

Both the Gita and the psalmist attempt to express in words the magnitude of God. Consider also a portion of the *Sophia of Jesus Christ*, a gnostic manuscript among those found at Nagaa Hammadi, Egypt, in 1945. While outside the canon of Christian scripture, and later denounced as heretical, the Sophia (wisdom) of Jesus Christ offers what might be considered supporting evidence for the idea of the cosmic and eternal Christ—without beginning or end:

---

39. Richard Rohr, "One Sacred World," Center for Action and Contemplation, March 26, 2015, *https://cac.org/one-sacred-world-2015-03-26/*.

40. Bhagavad Gita, 10:20, 185.

41. Bhagavad Gita, 10:25, 186.

42. Bhagavad Gita, 10:31, 187.

43. Bhagavad Gita, 10:32, 187.

44. Bhagavad Gita, 10:39, 189.

45. Bhagavad Gita, 10:42, 189.

> The Savior said: "He Who Is is ineffable. No principle knew him, no authority, no subjection, nor any creature from the foundation of the world until now, except he alone, and anyone to whom he wants to make revelation through him who is from First Light. From now on, I am the Great Savior. For he is immortal and eternal. Now he is eternal, having no birth; for everyone who has birth will perish. He is unbegotten, having no beginning; for everyone who has a beginning has an end. Since no one rules over him, he has no name; for whoever has a name [or human form] is the creation of another.[46]

This manuscript was considered gnostic and therefore denounced as heretical by orthodox Christianity. Perhaps it was merely too Eastern, too mystical for Western comfort. Sometimes you have to stand on the teetering edge of orthodoxy to find connections beyond your own tradition.

"Whatever You Do, Make It an Offering to Me," and the Science of Gratitude

A number of Bible verses instruct us to give thanks to the Lord always or to dedicate whatever we do to God. I confess I've always tended to read these as proscriptive: stay so busy giving thanks to God that you don't have time to do anything naughty. Such a reading yields a God who seeks to exhaust us and sets us up for shame when we bitch, moan, and carry on about life. Learning about the physiological benefits of gratitude has invited me to see these verses differently.

Researchers have found a causal link between sustained and high anxiety (which one could argue is fed by bitching, moaning, and carrying on) and increased inflammation in the body. High levels of inflammation in the body can weaken our immune system and increase our risk for physical illness. Chronic worry causes a lot of wear and tear inside our bodies.[47] So, because of the physical cost to being anxious all the time, it behooves us to find ways to reduce or even eliminate our anxiety.

---

46. Douglas M. Parrott, trans., "The Sophia of Jesus Christ," Early Christian Writings, accessed October 18, 2021, *http://www.earlychristianwritings.com/text/sophia.html.*

47. Nancy A. Melville, "Worry, Anxiety Tied to Increased Inflammation," Medscape, April 7, 2020, *https://www.medscape.com/viewarticle/928287*; N. Vogelzangs et al., "Anxiety Disorders and Inflammation in a Large Adult Cohort," *Translational Psychiatry* 3, no. 4 (2013): e249, *https://www.ncbi.nlm.nih.gov/pmc/articles/PMC3641413/*; Jennifer C. Felger, "Imaging the Role of Inflammation in Mood and Anxiety-Related Disorders," *Current Neuropharmacology* 16, no. 5 (2018): 533–58, *https://www.ncbi.nlm.nih.gov/pmc/articles/PMC5997866/*.

Enter the practice of gratitude. Researchers have looked at what happens when people spend as little as five minutes a day engaged in the practice of gratitude journaling. Over a two-month period, they found this practice lowered stress and improved sleep. A gratitude journaling practice lowered the hematological markers in the blood for inflammation, including the hemoglobin A1C, which is "associated with risk of heart failure, heart attacks, diabetes, chronic kidney disease, various cancers, and death."[48] If you are curious to learn more about the science of gratitude, check out the work of Dr. Robert Emmons, a professor of psychology at the University of California, Davis. Emmons has written or contributed to a number of books about gratitude and has undertaken an interesting study about gratitude and God.

Thinking about the physiological benefits of gratitude has helped me read certain parts of scripture in a new way. I want to share two passages. The first is probably familiar to you: "This is the day that the Lord has made; let us rejoice and be glad in it" (Ps. 118:24 ESV). The second is from the first letter to the Thessalonians (5:18): "Give thanks in all circumstances; for this is the will of God in Christ Jesus for you."

What if, instead of being directive, these scriptures are actually a compassionate prescription for our mental and physical health? Rejoice and be glad in this day, and you'll be doing your body and brain a favor. Give thanks in all circumstances because it'll help your body and brain stay healthy, and health is what God wills and wishes for you. Pretty different, yes? In that spirit, consider the following verses.

> Whatever I am offered in devotion with a pure heart . . . I accept with joy. Whatever you do, make it an offering to me—the food you eat, the sacrifices you make, the help you give, even your suffering. In this way you will be freed from the bondage of karma, and from its results both pleasant and painful. Then, firm in renunciation and yoga, with your heart free, you will come to me.[49] (Bhagavad Gita 9:26–28)

The Gita promises a free heart and freedom from "the bondage of karma" (remember that karma refers to mental activity as well as physical action), the removal of obstacles in the path to union with the divine.

---

48. Jeremy Adam Smith et al., eds., *The Gratitude Project: How the Science of Thankfulness Can Rewire Our Brains for Resilience, Optimism, and the Greater Good* (Oakland, CA: New Harbinger Publications, 2020), 44.

49. Bhagavad Gita, 176–77.

In Paul's letter to the Colossians (3:1–17), he counsels them to remember that because of the resurrected Christ, in whose risen life they now share, they should set their minds on "things that are above" and not on earthly concerns. "Put to death, therefore," says Paul, everything that is earthly. He describes those earthly things as fornication, evil desire, greed, anger, malice, and so on. He advises the Corinthians to clothe themselves instead with the virtues of love, compassion, and patience. He tells them to sing to God with gratitude in their hearts, and whatever they do "in word or deed, do everything in the name of the Lord Jesus, giving thanks to God the Father through him."

Romans 12:1–2 NCV echoes the offering language of the Gita:

> So brothers and sisters, since God has shown us great mercy, I beg you to offer your lives as a living sacrifice to him. Your offering must be only for God and pleasing to him, which is the spiritual way for you to worship. Do not be shaped by this world; instead be changed within by a new way of thinking. Then you will be able to decide what God wants for you; you will know what is good and pleasing to him and what is perfect.

It's helpful to read "perfect" as "whole, complete, fully developed, fully enlightened," which are valid translations of the Greek.[50] Being filled with gratitude is the way God intended for us to move through life. When we are filled with gratitude, we are whole and complete.

Easwaran observes that "everything is to be done and given and endured and enjoyed for the sake of the Lord in all, not for ourselves. . . . In practical terms, it means that awareness will be integrated down to the deepest recesses of the unconscious, which is precisely the significance of the word *yoga*."[51]

In contemporary Christian circles, Benedictine monk Brother David Steindl-Rast has long written about the practice of gratitude. He finds the practice has a positive impact far beyond an individual's enjoyment of a life in God and says that "grateful individuals live in a way that leads to the kind of society human beings long for."[52] The practice of gratitude is the antidote for some of the very sins Paul listed in Colossians 3: through grateful living, we become "aware that there is enough for all" and can release the sense of scarcity that drives us to greed.[53] "Grateful living," he explains, "is the awareness that

---

50. Strong's Greek Concordance, No. 5046.

51. Bhagavad Gita, 55–56.

52. Smith, *The Gratitude Project*, 197.

53. Smith, *The Gratitude Project*, 198.

we stand on holy ground—always—in touch with Mystery."[54] If we are always standing on holy ground, in touch with the mystery of God, then giving thanks in all circumstances becomes a way to keep our feet planted in holiness—in divine wholeness, which is our birthright.

Tapas and the Passion of Jesus

Have you ever had the experience of creating something and in the process lost track of time and the world around you? The process of bringing forth something new requires our focus. It is all-consuming and yet satisfying because something of us lives on in that which we created. In return for our expenditure, we get the privilege of living beyond the confines of our physical selves. Through the book or poem or painting we create, something of us gets to interact with people we will personally never meet in our flesh. Of course, this same "living beyond ourselves" happens also as the result of the process of creating a new human life.

In some infinitesimal way, when we laser-beam our focus during the creative process, when we step free of the chains of *chronos* time, when we find ourselves falling in love with or delighting in what we are creating, we mimic God the Creator whose image we bear. In the Genesis creation story, God creates in peristaltic sound waves: Let there be light; let there be a dome called sky; let waters gather together and dry land appear; let the earth put forth vegetation; and so on. God pronounces the product of each wave good.

Genesis 2:3 says that when all was done, God set time apart for the purpose of rest, blessed that time, and then rested from the divine work. The Greek for "work" is εργον [*ergon*], from which the word *erg* is drawn. In physics, an erg is a unit of work or energy. Work expends energy, and energy produces heat.

This understanding leads us to the yogic word *tapas*, which is derived from the Sanskrit root word *tap,* which means to burn, blaze, shine, suffer pain, or consume heat. *Tapas* is the internal fire in a person that is stoked by effort, zeal, intense concentration, austerity, and self-discipline.[55] It is the kind of intensity of purpose Jesus had as he moved toward Jerusalem in his final days. In Matthew 16, Jesus tells Peter that Peter is the rock on which the church will be built. Presumably, Peter felt honored, even if he didn't understand exactly what Jesus meant. And yet mere sentences later in Matthew's account (vv. 21–23), Jesus

54. Smith, *The Gratitude Project*, 199.

55. "Tapas," The Yoga Sanctuary, accessed October 18, 2021, https://www.theyogasanctuary.biz/tapas/.

snaps at his favored disciple. "Get behind me, Satan!" he says to Peter rebukingly. Why? Because Peter's unwillingness or inability to grasp the mission of Jesus was a stumbling block. Jesus blazed with *tapas* for his mission and would not be deterred from it. We might say he had a *passion* for carrying out his calling.

The ancient sage Patanjali offered a Yoga Sutra (2.1) that speaks of the role of *tapas* in achieving yoga, or union with God: "Austerity, study, and the dedication of the fruits of one's work to God: these are the preliminary steps toward yoga."[56] The Sanskrit for "austerity" is *tapas*, and in this sutra, expressing it in English is problematic. One translator says the only other English words available are "mortification" and "discipline," and unfortunately, the negative connotation those words carry in our language renders an aphorism that is puritanical and harsh.[57] The truer meaning of the aphorism is a self-discipline that allows one to conserve and focus the energy toward a goal, the goal of union with God. It is a self-discipline or austerity that is joyful and life-giving. The translator says, "True austerity, in the Hindu understanding of the word, is not a process of fanatical self-punishment but of quiet and sane control."[58] It is a passion that is harnessed and focused for a purpose.

In scripture, the Greek word παθημα [*pathéma*][59] means both "passion" and "suffering." Of the word's sixteen occurrences in the New Testament, only two employ "passion" to mean sinful desire.[60] The rest all translate as suffering.[61] In either case, the word describes the ability to feel strong emotion. Passion or *tapas* is a quality humans have long assigned to God, in addition to recognizing it as part of the human condition.

The Rig Veda is a collection of Sanskrit hymns of praise estimated to have been written between 1500 and 1200 BCE. This places it earlier than the compilation of the book of Genesis. Easwaran says that *tapas* is an "ardent, one-pointed, and self-transcending passion," and the Vedic texts "revere it as an unsurpassable creative force."[62] According to Easwaran, the Rig Veda says that the cosmos was born from the *tapas* of God.[63] There are curious similarities

---

56. Prabhavananda and Isherwood, *How to Know God*, 99.

57. Prabhavananda and Isherwood, *How to Know God*, 100.

58. Prabhavananda and Isherwood, *How to Know God*, 102.

59. Strong's 3804 and 3806.

60. "3804. pathéma," Bible Hub, accessed October 18, 2021, *https://biblehub.com/greek/3804.htm*.

61. "3958. paschó," Bible Hub, accessed October 18, 2021, *https://biblehub.com/greek/3958.htm*.

62. Upanishads, 34.

63. Upanishads, 34.

between a creation hymn[64] in the Rig Veda and the opening verses (1:1–7) of the book of Genesis.

In the hymn, the Rig Veda describes an unfathomed depth of water. Genesis describes a fathomless deep. The Rig Veda indicates there was no sign to divide the day from the night. In Genesis, separating the two was one of God's first acts and was the purpose of creating light. The Rig Veda describes a formless void, chaotic and concealed in darkness. Genesis says that "the earth was a formless void and darkness covered the face of the deep" (v. 2).

The Rig Veda hymn speaks of divine desire, calling it "the primal seed and germ of Spirit." Although Genesis does not speak explicitly about creation being driven by God's desire, the narrator implies it when after each creative wave God "saw that it was good." God, being God, *desires* to create something good and is satisfied when such is done. It is further implied after God makes the Adamah—the earth creature—and says, "It is not good that the man should be alone; I will make him a helper as his partner" (2:18). God's *desire* for goodness and completeness is inherent in creation.

If the first law of thermodynamics[65] holds true of God, then God's expenditure of energy in the creating of the universe was not a loss of energy but a transfer of energy from God to creation. God spent something of Godself to create the world. That "something" was not lost but appeared in new form: the created order. In an outpouring of love and desire, God chose to take a portion of Godself and manifest it as creation.

The Way We Pray

For centuries, Christians have used their bodies to engage in prayer. Since the Enlightenment, and the mind–body separatism posited by René Descartes (1596–1650), our prayer practice seems to have gradually lodged more comfortably in the intellect and become less physical. Various religious orders, among them the Ignatians, Dominicans, and Carmelites, call us back to enlisting the body in prayer, as does yoga, which in fact some orders use as a tool to prepare and quiet the mind for prayer.

In the summer of 1971, Edward B. Fiske, an education writer with a master's in theology, interviewed nuns, priests, and brothers at an ecumenical yoga

64. Ralph T. H. Griffith, "Book 10, hymn 129, verses 1–7," sacred-texts.com, accessed October 18, 2021, *https://www.sacred-texts.com/hin/rigveda/rv10129.htm*.

65. "Introduction to Thermodynamics," Lumen, accessed October 18, 2021, *https://courses.lumenlearning.com/boundless-chemistry/chapter/introduction-to-thermodynamics/*.

retreat. They had gathered to hear the teachings of Swami Satchidananda, an Indian Hindu monk, who in 1966 had founded the Integral Yoga Institute in New York. His belief was that the principles underlying yoga could be applied readily to all religions and that "the purpose of all religions is to teach [the practitioner] to give [oneself] to God. . . . The Yoga discipline leads to purity and a selfless attitude that helps make this possible."[66] Giving oneself to God is what Christians seek to do in prayer.

At the retreat Fiske covered for the *New York Times*, celebration of the Holy Eucharist was offered alongside the study and practice of yoga. He interviewed a Discalced Carmelite nun who explained that practicing yoga deepened her prayer life by relaxing and integrating her body and mind and by helping her transcend the senses.

Parallels have been drawn between the breath practices of the Hesychasts and pranayama, or yogic breathing techniques. "Hesychast" is from the Greek ησυχαζω [*hésuchazó*], meaning "to be still, at rest, to be quiet, or to live peaceably."[67] Inspired by Jesus's instruction to pray to the Father in secret (Matt. 6:5–6), Hesychasts began in the early centuries of Christianity, among the Desert Fathers, to turn inward in their prayer practice. They employed the breath to pray the Jesus prayer: on the inhale, the words "Lord Jesus Christ, Son of God"; on the exhale, the words "have mercy on me a sinner."[68] In *Jesus in the Lotus*, Russill Paul finds compelling evidence for the influence of yogic practice on the early Hesychasts, who later became part of the Eastern Orthodox tradition of Christianity.[69] In *Sophia Rising*, Monette Chilson likewise highlights a strong historic connection between yogic practice and Hesychasm.[70] Tempering their findings is Eastern Orthodox bishop and theologian Kallistos Ware, who in an essay on the Jesus Prayer wrote:

> Striking parallels exist between the physical techniques recommended by the Byzantine Hesychasts and those employed in Hindu Yoga and in Sufism. How far are the similarities the result of the mere coincidence, of an independent

66. Edward B. Fiske, "Priests and Nuns Discover Yoga Enhances Grasp of Faith," *New York Times*, July 2, 1971, 35, *https://www.nytimes.com/1971/07/02/archives/priests-and-nuns-discover-yoga-enhances-grasp-of-faith-priests-and.html.*

67. Strong's Greek Concordance, No. 2270.

68. Bishop Kallistos-Ware, "Jesus Prayer—Breathing Exercises," Jesus Prayer—Breathing Exercises, accessed October 18, 2021, *https://www.orthodoxprayer.org/Articles_files/Ware-7%20Breathing%20Exercises.html.*

69. Paul, *Jesus in the Lotus*, 49.

70. Chilson, *Sophia Rising*, 96–98.

> though analogous development in two separate traditions? If there is a direct relation between Hesychasm and Sufism—which side has been borrowing from the other? Here is a fascinating field for research, although the evidence is perhaps too fragmentary to permit any definite conclusion.[71]

Ware goes on to caution that while there are certainly similarities between yogic techniques and the Jesus Prayer, there is a key difference: the "distinctively Christian content of the Prayer. The essential point in the Jesus Prayer is not the act of repetition in itself, not how we sit or breathe, but to whom we speak; and in this instance the words are addressed unambiguously to the Incarnate Saviour Jesus Christ, Son of God and Son of Mary."[72]

It is tempting to make Jesus into a yogi, with his habit of withdrawing and going inward to pray. Whether Jesus saw himself as a yogi and whether his followers saw him as such are two very different and unanswerable matters. A curious hint in favor of the latter is the preponderance of Coptic, Byzantine, and Eastern Orthodox iconography depicting Jesus with his hands in unmistakable *mudras*. A mudra is a ritual or symbolic gesture, usually made with the hands. Mudras have a role in Indian classical dance as well as religion. In yoga, mudras are used to facilitate the flow of energy between the chakras, or energy centers in the body.

Four to five centuries before Jesus, in writings by Aristophanes, Xenophon, and Plato, the Greek word υποκριτησ [*hupokrités*] for "hypocrite" arose. [73] In Matthew 6:5–6 Jesus said: "And whenever you pray, do not be like the hypocrites; for they love to stand and pray in the synagogues and at the street corners, so that they may be seen by others. Truly I tell you, they have received their reward. But whenever you pray, go into your room and shut the door and pray to your Father who is in secret; and your Father who sees in secret will reward you."

The Greek υποκριτησ [*hupokrités*] also means "actor" or "stage-player." This meaning accords with Jesus's injunction not to "go onstage" at the local synagogue or street corner to perform your piety for all to see.[74] In verse 5, the reward—in Greek, the μισθοσ [*misthos*], or "payment for hire"[75]—of a hypocrite is not union with the Father but the accolades of their peers. As actors, they have hired themselves out for this pay.

---

71. Kallistos-Ware, "Jesus Prayer—Breathing Exercises."

72. Kallistos-Ware, "Jesus Prayer—Breathing Exercises."

73. William F. Arndt and F. Wilbur Gingrich, *A Greek-English Lexicon of the New Testament and Other Early Christian Literature*, 2nd ed. (Chicago: University of Chicago Press, 1979), 845.

74. Strong's Greek Concordance, No. 5273.

75. Strong's Greek Concordance, No. 3408.

In verse 6, the Greek word for "reward"—namely, God's reward to the one praying—is different: αποδιδωμι [*apodidómi*] means to answer one's expectation, to restore, to render back to, or to requite—to respond to or to return one's love and affection.[76] Unlike "reward" in the previous verse, this reward is not transactional but relational. God does not respond transactionally as a divine vending machine into which we plug nickels with a flourish. God responds by upholding God's side of a covenantal relationship.

One more note on the Greek helps open this verse to a yogic understanding: in verse 6 the Father is described as being and seeing "in secret." Another valid translation for κρυπτοσ [*kruptos*] is "hidden or concealed."[77] If God is "in us," then God is hidden or concealed from view. The way to meet God in prayer is thus to go within.

Easwaran describes a similar path toward union with God: practicing *nishkama karma*. To do this is to work without selfish motive or selfish desire. One might say that a person practicing *nishkama karma* is acting purely, without hypocrisy, with no expectation of reward or recompense.[78] The key word here is *selfish*. The Bhagavad Gita doesn't disparage desire itself, for human desire can lead us to do great things. It is the "fierce, compulsive craving for personal satisfaction"—desire run amok—that is harmful.[79] Action free of selfish desire serves to purify the mind, says Easwaran,[80] and the Gita illustrates this: "You have the right to work, but never to the fruit of work. You should never engage in action for the sake of reward. . . . Those who are motivated only by desire or the fruits of action are miserable, for they are constantly anxious about the results of what they do."[81] "Do not be anxious about anything," Paul told the Christians at Philippi (4:6–7), but "in everything by prayer and supplication with thanksgiving let your requests be made known to God." God's response will be "the peace . . . which surpasses all understanding."

Theological Meeting Places Yet to Be Explored

Sometimes you meet someone and there is a flash of connection—two souls each recognizing something kindred in the other. If you are traveling or live in

76. Strong's Greek Concordance, No. 591.

77. Strong's Greek Concordance, No. 2927.

78. Bhagavad Gita, 52.

79. Bhagavad Gita, 52.

80. Bhagavad Gita, 53.

81. Bhagavad Gita, 2.47–49, 94.

an urban area, you may never see the other person again. Even so, you go on with your day knowing that in that moment, that one brief moment, you were privileged to partake in an encounter that was pregnant with the possibility of something more. It is uplifting, especially if you are someone who regards possibilities as riches.

Likewise, a wealth of encounters between yogic philosophy and progressive, mystical Christian theology are yet to be explored. Is there a parallel between the awakening of *prana* (life force or energy) and being filled with the Holy Spirit? How might the *yama*s and *niyamas*—the ethical guidelines of yoga—converse with the Ten Commandments of Christianity? What relationship might there be between the seven chakras (the energy centers in the body) of yogic philosophy and how the seven deadly sins manifest in the human person? How can recent discoveries in scientific disciplines like neuroscience and quantum physics expand the common ground for discussion between Christianity and yogic philosophy? Others have written, and written well, about some of these. Much more remains to be explored. "I dwell in possibility," wrote Emily Dickinson. Possibility was where Dickinson found paradise. [82]

82. Emily Dickinson, "I Dwell in Possibility," in *The Poems of Emily Dickinson*, ed. R. W. Franklin (Cambridge, MA: Harvard University Press, 1999).

4

PREPARING FOR YOGA IN *YOUR* CHURCH

You could not step twice into the same river; for other waters are ever flowing on to you.

—*Heraclitus of Ephesus (540 BC–480 BC), "On the Universe"*[1]

HAVE YOU EVER STOOD AT THE CONFLUENCE of two rivers and watched the power of moving water meeting moving water? Even if the water looks calm at the meeting place, beneath the surface two very different sets of currents from two very different ecosystems are encountering each other, spinning and twirling together like otters before they become a single body of water. Hydrologists explain that "river confluences are complex hydrodynamic environments where convergence of incoming flows produces complicated patterns of fluid motion, including the development of large-scale turbulence structures."[2] That means if you are crossing a river, especially near the confluence with another water source, you need to be alert to your footing. You need to be nimble and agile, be prepared to get wet, and have a plan for how to exit the current safely if you get swept away. If you are a hike master or expedition leader in charge of moving a group of people safely across a river, you need to be especially attentive. This is a good image to bear in mind as you invite your parish into the confluence to explore the meeting place of Christianity and yoga.

The first portion of this chapter regards preparing the congregation to receive, embrace, and participate in this new ministry of yoga in the worship space. In chapter 6 you'll find stories from Episcopal churches that are already offering this ministry. Let their successes and failures help guide you. The

1. "River and Environmental Quotations," National Wild and Scenic Rivers System, accessed October 18, 2021, *https://www.rivers.gov/quotations.php*.

2. George Constantinescu et al., "Structure of Turbulent Flow at a River Confluence with Momentum and Velocity Ratios Close to 1: Insight Provided by an Eddy-Resolving Numerical Solution," *Water Resources Research* 47, no. 5 (2011): *https://agupubs.onlinelibrary.wiley.com/doi/full/10.1029/2010WR010018*.

second portion of this chapter regards the more practical preparations: considerations of space, setting, advertising, finding the right teachers, and so on.

I am a teacher at heart, so my counsel is to begin preparing your congregation by teaching them, not about yoga but about sacred space. Many of us Episcopalians like to think we are progressive—theologically expansive and dynamic thinkers—and your congregation may reflect that self-perception. Even if they do, take care not to discount the concerns of the quiet traditionalists, who may harbor misconceptions about what yoga is and question why the practice of it is appropriate in a Christian worship space.

Where precisely you start in your teaching will depend on the culture and context of your parish. Is your church dwindling in size and struggling to reach potential new members? Is the parish interested in becoming more involved in the surrounding community but has little sense of how to do that? Do you and your parish want to go deeper in your spiritual practices of prayer, contemplation, study, and worship and wonder what the best approach might be? Are you fresh out of ideas (and guest speakers) for the Sunday after-worship adult formation hour? If Yoga in the Church can be offered as a possible response to an articulated need or desire, it's much more likely to be received well than if it simply drops out of the sky and lands in warrior II pose on the carpet in the nave.

The suggestions for teaching that follow are just that—suggestions. Choose from them to craft an approach that will best speak to what you identify as the hunger in your parish. If you skipped over chapters 1 and 2, go back and read them with the intent of harvesting material you can use in teaching your congregation about yoga. The extent to which you take your time building curiosity about and support for Yoga in the Church will dictate how broadly your congregation embraces this new ministry.

That's Right, You're Standing on It

I first encountered an iconostasis in the 1980s when I was living in an Alaskan village off the road system. The area had been occupied by Indigenous tribes for millennia. In the eighteenth century, Russian fur traders arrived and, not long after, Russian Orthodox missionary priests. In modern times, many of the villagers claimed a Native Alaskan and Russian lineage, and a charming little wooden Russian Orthodox church stood in a place of prominence on a cliff overlooking the bay. Priests were in short supply, so the village received a priestly visit only once a year. The father would arrive by bush plane and spend the next day or two hearing confessions, offering worship services and the Holy Eucharist, and perhaps performing baptisms or a wedding.

One year I attended worship. It was the first time I had been inside the historic structure and the first time I had seen the ornate wall of icons behind the altar that separated the priest-only holy space from the main body or nave of the church. Every now and again the priest would disappear back there and then reemerge to continue with the hours-long service. The iconostasis separated and set apart the holy of holies from the worshipers in the main body of the church, evoking the layout of the ancient Jerusalem temple. The priest, in his role as mediator between the people and God, was the only one allowed to go "behind the curtain."

We don't have a similar theology of space in an Episcopal church—formally, that is. Practically speaking, I have witnessed a reluctance among laypersons (altar guilds notwithstanding) to approach the altar, to touch it, or to stand behind it in the place customarily reserved for the priest. I want to distinguish here between reverence and reluctance. The former is good; the latter, less so. If we are to embrace the priesthood of all believers, timidity isn't healthy or helpful. The typical church architecture promotes the unhelpful separation of priest and people, with the altar often on a raised platform many feet distant from the rows of pews bolted to the floor. In my parish, I have looked for opportunities to teach around these physical constraints and promote the idea that while the whole church may "belong" to God in one sense, *the whole church also belongs to all its people.* The priest in her unique role may be set apart, but she is set apart *from within* the body of the people, and all approach God as equals.

When children in my parish complete their first communion instruction, they are invited to stand around the altar with the priest for the celebration of the Holy Eucharist. They stand on footstools so the congregation gets to see something more than the tops of their little heads and so they can see the congregation. I invite them to make the gestures of the eucharistic prayer with me, imprinting their bodies in some small way, I hope, with an embodied and priestly piety. Whenever we have a family service, we invite children to stand around the altar with the priest. Children are always called forward at baptisms so they can witness that sacrament up close, and in pre-pandemic times I even invited them to plunge their hands into the water with me.

Adults are likewise invited to get up from their pews and come forward to lay hands on someone marking a significant life occasion to help bless them. Often there are so many people it creates a big and holy scrum. At the communion rail, young acolytes who feel so called are invited to join the priest in laying a hand on those parishioners who ask for a blessing—with the parishioner's permission, of course. There are many ways to teach and model for your parish that worship involves everyone and that every square foot of real estate in the church (and beyond the doors too) is holy ground. You don't need to wait for a yoga ministry to begin teaching this.

Every parish—including my own—has people who are resolute in their conviction that if yoga is to be in the church it should be in the basement or the parish hall or the room where twelve-step groups hold their meetings. This conviction misses the whole point: Yoga is an act of worship. Yoga deepens our worship of the very same God we meet on Sunday mornings. It belongs, therefore, in the worship space. There is also something deeply healing for people about being in a worship space and using their bodies to seek union with God. Inevitably, after a Yoga in the Church workshop, someone approaches with tears in their eyes and explains how they had felt judged or wounded by a Christian church so left it but have missed it terribly. To be welcomed back into the worship space in this new way is, for some, a very emotional homecoming. That alone should be enough to commend it, for as our prayer book reminds us, we are, after all, a church whose mission it is "to restore all people to unity with God and each other in Christ."[3]

Read with your congregation the story of Moses and the burning bush from Exodus chapter 3. They already know the takeaway line in verse 5: Then [God] said, "Come no closer! Remove the sandals from your feet, for the place on which you are standing is holy ground." What made it holy, I believe, was that God and man encountered each other there. Wherever we stand when we encounter God, that place becomes holy ground.

In her book *Christ in Evolution*, scientist and theologian Ilia Delio cites Pierre Teilhard de Chardin in suggesting that the role of the Christian is, in cooperation with God, *to actually make* holy ground. Teilhard de Chardin

> emphasized that the role of the Christian is to divinize the world in Jesus Christ, to "christify" the world by our actions, by immersing ourselves in the world, plunging our hands, we might say, into the soil of the earth and touching the roots of life. In [de Chardin's] *Divine Milieu* he wrote, "There is nothing profane here below for those who know how to see." The world, he claimed, is like a crystal lamp illumined from within by the light of Christ. For those who can see, Christ shines in this diaphanous universe, through the cosmos and in matter.[4]

---

3. *The Book of Common Prayer*, 855.

4. Delio, *Christ in Evolution*, 139.

There are those who may concede that the entire planet may be sheathed in holy ground but a church is *more* holy because an Episcopal bishop consecrated it as such. What does your diocesan bishop have to say about this? Can she or he be an ally to you as you seek to bring yoga into your church worship space?

In "A Liturgy for the Opening of a New Congregation," the Episcopal Church acknowledges that holy ground is not limited to the nave, chancel, and sanctuary of a church and that consecrating a space for worship does not take other uses off the table: "This rite is designed for use by a church planting team or new congregation, as it begins worship in a facility such as a school, nursing home, 'storefront' or other secular space. With adaptation it could be used in a variety of other situations, such as the initial gathering of a retreat group in a hotel. It anticipates regular but not exclusive use of the room or building for worship purposes."[5]

An interesting way to invite your congregation to enlarge their definition of holy ground and the use of consecrated space is to read together Sara Miles's book *Take This Bread*. Miles found her way to St. Gregory of Nyssa Episcopal Church in San Francisco, a congregation noted for its inclusivity and innovative worship style. The church had just taken delivery of a gorgeous custom-made $6,000 altar, inscribed with biblical verses that reminded worshipers of the universal welcome of Jesus.[6] As Miles worshiped at that altar week after week and was fed by the Holy Eucharist, she became increasingly aware of (and uncomfortable with) the dichotomy of the city in which she lived: a food-obsessed "foodie" populace with neighborhoods such as the Mission District also displayed abject poverty for those with the eyes to see. She began to get a vision: that St. Gregory's new altar should be used as a grocery distribution station for the poor, putting a new spin on Jesus's command to "feed my sheep."

Miles had a holy idea, but the people of St. Gregory's did not embrace her idea at first. She spoke to the priest, who worried such a ministry would polarize the parish. She wrote to the vestry and pitched her idea to the staff, outreach committee, and parish. The outreach committee chair explained that, being new, Miles knew nothing about church volunteer burnout and that their congregation was busy enough already. Some objections had to do with "strangers" in "our church." The staff was similarly unsupportive, with reactions ranging from "'Over my dead body' to 'When hell freezes over.'"[7] Miles did not give up, and eventually, the church conceded to let her give the food pantry idea a

5. *The Book of Occasional Services 2003* (New York, NY: Church Publishing, 2004), 244.

6. Sara Miles, *Take This Bread: A Radical Conversion* (New York: Ballantine Books, 2007), 111.

7. Miles, *Take This Bread*, 114.

try. That was nearly twenty years ago. The Food Pantry at St. Gregory of Nyssa Episcopal Church is still there and has grown from feeding 35 families a week to feeding 400. We can learn something from Miles's story about seeking to introduce to the church a new way of being the church.

Expanding Our Definition of "Worship"

In an adult formation hour, ask your parish to define the word *worship*. Offer no further instruction or prompt. Let their input flow freely. Record their answers. When all who care to share have done so, go back and highlight some common themes. Circle back and check in with the group to see if they want to add anything else before you move on.

Highlight those bits of input that regard using our bodies. For example, if someone said, "Worship is bringing our bodies, voices, hearts, and minds to God and to each other," circle that. Now read the Greek definition of "worship" from the New Testament: προσκυϖεω [*proskuneó*] means to do reverence to by inclining the body toward the person or object and kissing the ground (or their hand, or the hem of their garment). Inclining the body might be a bow, or kneeling, or prostrating oneself, the body face-down on the ground.[8] The New Testament writers understood worship to be a very physical act.

In the following Gospel passages, Matthew and Mark employ the Greek προσκυϖεω [*proskuneó*], even though the NRSV does not translate it consistently as "worship." All emphases are mine.

> On entering the house, they saw the child with Mary his mother; and they *knelt down and paid him homage*. Then, opening their treasure chests, they offered him gifts of gold, frankincense, and myrrh. (Matt. 2:11)
>
> But [the Canaanite woman] came and *knelt before* [Jesus], saying, "Lord, help me." (Matt. 15:25)
>
> So the slave *fell on his knees before* [the king], saying, "Have patience with me, and I will pay you everything.: (Matt. 18:26)
>
> When [the Gerasene demoniac] saw Jesus from a distance, he ran and *bowed down before* him; and he shouted at the top of his voice, "What have you to do with me, Jesus, Son of the Most High God? I adjure you by God, do not torment me." (Mark 5:6–7)

8. "4352. proskuneó," Bible Hub, accessed October 18, 2021, *https://biblehub.com/greek/4352.htm*; Arndt and Gingrich, *A Greek-English Lexicon of the New Testament and Other Early Christian Literature*, 716–17.

> And they began saluting [Jesus], "Hail, King of the Jews!" They struck his head with a reed, spat upon him, and *knelt down in homage to* him. (Mark 15:18–19)

Kneeling down, falling down, kneeling before, falling on the knees, bowing down, kneeling down in homage—you get the idea. If a space is set aside and consecrated for worship, it's safe to assume the New Testament writers knew we'd be moving our bodies in some way. Even so, depictions of early Christians moving their bodies in worship or dancing ecstatically are sparse. Why? Perhaps it is because the earliest Jesus followers were by necessity surreptitious worshipers, crowding themselves into private homes and conducting rites in the catacombs. It didn't leave much room for a dance floor, and liturgical processions didn't become normative until the fourth century and the legalization of Christianity (and subsequently, the declaration of it as the official religion of the Roman Empire). Once we moved out of the shadow of persecution, we could stretch our legs a little, so to speak.

Our Jewish ancestors in faith certainly moved their bodies as part of worship. Consider Psalm 150:

> Praise the LORD!
> 　Praise God in his sanctuary;
> praise him in his mighty firmament!
> Praise him for his mighty deeds;
> 　praise him according to his surpassing greatness!
> Praise him with trumpet sound;
> 　praise him with lute and harp!
> Praise him with tambourine and dance;
> 　praise him with strings and pipe!
> Praise him with clanging cymbals;
> 　praise him with loud clashing cymbals!
> Let everything that breathes praise the LORD!
> 　Praise the LORD!

It is hard to read this psalm as one written to a people who sat still and siloed in neat rows of pews. "Praise him with tambourine and dance!" That's clearly a full-body experience of worship.

At the close of chapter 2, I spoke about the Christian tendency toward frozen chosen-ness. It bears some discussion in the parish: Do folks feel a twinge of embarrassment about this label (that's good), or do they proudly claim it as a moniker or tagline (not so good)? Even if your congregation lands solidly in the latter camp, there still may be an opening wide enough to permit yoga to come in to the life of the parish. That opening needs only be as wide as a child. Children love and benefit from yoga just like adults, and their very innocence and enthusiasm are effective at softening our defenses. Perhaps your church might start with Yoga in the Church workshops for children and youth.

Identifying and Teaching to the Misconceptions

Yoga Journal and the professional organization Yoga Alliance regularly surveys yoga practitioners, yoga studio owners, yoga teachers, and nonpractitioners. Their report can provide a sense of how many people practice yoga in your part of the country. The report also identifies the barriers that inhibit people from starting a yoga practice. Those who've never tried yoga say they don't know if it's right for them and they don't know how to get started.[9] Even among practitioners, 40 percent believe yoga is for really flexible people, and 54 percent believe it is for athletes.[10]

Be alert to these concerns as you begin to explore with your congregation the idea of bringing yoga into the church. Those who practice yoga know that it can be safely and effectively adapted to any body type or level of ability, including those differently abled who rely on walkers or wheelchairs. At St. John's, our workshops are for everyone, including those who want to come in street clothes, sit in the pews, and listen. Also be mindful that the same pastoral sensitivity you extend to participants in other ministries is all the more important with yoga. Many of us have tenuous relationships with our bodies, ranging from distrust to outright hate. Assure people that they need not own Spandex in order to practice yoga.

We don't have a dress code for our Yoga in the Church workshops and have found that everyone shows up reasonably garbed without any instruction from us. We do advise attendees to wear layers, because high-ceilinged worship spaces can be drafty. God has no need for us to be human peacocks when practicing yoga in a church, and if we have such a need to be on display in a worship space, it invites self-examination of our motives. Any kind of clothing that

9. "2016 Yoga in America Study," Ipsos Public Affairs, January 2016, *https://www.yogaalliance.org/Portals/0/2016%20Yoga%20in%20America%20Study%20RESULTS.pdf, 41.*

10. Ibid, 26.

allows free movement and promotes comfort is acceptable. Each human body is exquisitely beautiful to God, the maker of us all.

As you seek to uncover your parish's misconceptions about yoga, consider a survey. Make it an anonymous one to encourage honest responses, and make it short and sweet. Explore areas of inquiry such as these:

- Have you tried yoga? If yes, do you practice regularly? What do you like about your practice?
- If no, why not? What barriers do you imagine or did you encounter?
- Do you wish for more spiritual depth in your life of faith? Would you like to have more tools to deepen your prayer practice? Tools to mediate anxiety?
- Do you think the practice of yoga is at odds with being a Christian?
- Are you curious to know about yogic philosophy and how it could shed light on Christian scripture and theology?

The answers you receive will help you discover the pulse of your parish and help you decide on a starting place in your teaching. If you feel ill-equipped to teach about the history, philosophy, and practice of yoga, worry not. Your community likely has people who can help. If you are in or close to a college town, contact the college's religious studies department and see if a faculty member could be invited to speak about Hinduism, Buddhism, and yogic philosophy. Even if there's not an institute of higher learning nearby, find and invite a scholar from your state university—or perhaps a university or college across the country—to speak to your parish by video conferencing platform.

Consider using Hindu-Christian Russill Paul's excellent and accessible book as a study aid for your parish. *Jesus in the Lotus: The Mystical Doorway between Christianity and Yogic Spirituality* makes a cogent and balanced argument for the compatibility of yoga and Christianity, and articulates how each can complement the other. Don't overlook the experts in your own parish. When I began offering Yoga in the Church workshops in my parish, a quiet, frail-looking older woman contacted me. She was a lifelong Episcopalian and a faithful member of the altar guild. I would not have pegged her for a yogi. "I am so glad you are doing this," she said. She went on to tell me she had studied the intersection of yoga and Christianity for nearly thirty-five years, starting in 1985 when she happened upon a yoga class taught by a very muscular woman. My parishioner—a fitness instructor herself—found the class dauntingly athletic. But something drew her back a second time and then a third. She was forty-nine at the time and decided she would do the best she could and not be concerned with "performance." She wrote, "For me, yoga was life-changing. Within a year or two, I achieved more from yoga physically, mentally, and spiritually than I ever thought possible. . . . The compelling pull of yoga (an art and philosophy) is the holistic approach of engaging mind, body, and spirit into everyday life. What is learned in class applies awareness and wisdom to daily living. . . . Yoga has enhanced and enriched my spiritual life, and I am so grateful for that." Now in her mid-eighties, my parishioner has given up the faster moving flows of vinyasa-style yoga but still practices Iyengar yoga, a school focused on structural alignment of the body in which poses are held for longer periods of time.

Find out who the devoted yogis are in your parish. Gather them for a conversation about their experience of yoga and whether and how it has informed their practice of Christianity. Are they able and willing to talk about any spiritual experiences they've had as a result of their yogic practice? Enlist them as resident experts, and invite the parish to a panel discussion featuring these yogis—their fellow parishioners. Such an approach not only normalizes the practice of yoga, it also can serve to lift up these parishioners as spiritual elders—or, at the least, people who are serious about their spiritual growth.

Once you find a suitable yoga teacher, offer an introductory "play-shop"—either a single event or a short series. Intentionally different from a workshop, a play-shop is a light-hearted opportunity to try out asanas, lose your balance, laugh, experiment, and call a pause so questions can be asked and addressed. A spirit of curiosity and self-discovery is the order of the day. Make it free of charge. Let it be an opportunity to introduce and demystify yoga. Go light on the philosophy, but do not abandon it altogether. Sirena will say more about how to create and offer a play-shop later in the chapter.

As you talk and write about bringing yoga into your church, be clear that this is an opt-in ministry and not something you're intending to add on to Sunday morning worship. You may think this is a point too evident to be worth mentioning, but know that anxiety about new things can impel people to make sweeping and inaccurate assumptions. As fun as it might be to imagine a Sunday morning church full of people balancing in tree pose while reciting the Nicene Creed, don't go there.

Set realistic expectations about what a Yoga in the Church ministry can and cannot do for the health of your church. Do your part to cultivate the right attitude: yoga is a ministry of spiritual growth, healing, and seed planting, not a panacea for a dwindling ASA (average Sunday attendance). One or more of the clergy in the parish should be involved as a co-teacher. This can be as simple as participating in the class and stepping forward to offer a short reflection or as complex as our Yoga in the Church model, where the clergyperson is a full co-teacher in every workshop. Engage a well-known lay leader or two (like vestry members) as workshop participants. The personal involvement of the clergy and lay leaders is very important to lend legitimacy to this or any ministry.

Acknowledge upfront that in the process of bringing something new into the worship space there will probably be bumps. I worked for one parish that welcomed the local Jewish community to hold weekly Shabbat services in the church. Beginning this ministry of sharing worship space was a generous, beautiful, and somewhat courageous move on the part of the rector. While most parishioners were proud to be members of a church that demonstrated such hospitality, some were less sure. They tolerated the shared use until something got broken or temporarily misplaced. Then bubbled up their resentment at "those people" in "our church," like the folks in Sara Miles's parish who were uneasy at sharing their worship space with a food pantry. Some careful attention can help avoid such conflicts, and if they do arise, an abundance of compassion can help smooth things. Several months after starting your Yoga in the Church ministry you might want to schedule a check-in with your altar guild (or any other group regularly in the worship space) and see if they feel you are being a good and respectful co-occupant.

Finding the Right Teacher

Finding the right yoga teacher is imperative to the success of your Yoga in the Church ministry. Have you ever experienced a yoga class in which you adored the teacher and wanted to come back as often as possible? On the flip side, have you experienced a yoga class with a teacher who completely turned you off—so much so that you never went back? The right teacher is both certified and qualified and will help ensure your workshop participants return again and again. Experience in teaching and public speaking is vital, as is a familiarity with—or at least a charitable attitude toward—Christianity. Certified yoga teachers hold either a 200-hour RYT (Registered Yoga Teacher) or 500-hour RYT, and this can be verified through certification websites such as Yoga Alliance (www.yogaalliance.org/). If you are not familiar with someone applying to teach, ask to see their certificate number or membership card, and ask for a copy of their insurance certificate to keep on file. Even though most churches are insured for injuries that take place on campus, a yoga teacher is also required to hold liability insurance for coverage against student injuries.

Look for a teacher who has at least one hundred hours of yoga teaching experience, as well as experience in creating, advertising, and leading workshops. The ideal teacher will not only be able to lead asanas but will also be well-versed in yogic philosophy and be able to speak compellingly in front of a class.

Not all yoga teacher training schools delve deeply into yogic philosophy. Some regard yoga primarily as exercise so concentrate on teaching the asanas and anatomy, to the detriment of the ancient and beautiful spiritual teachings. As you interview potential teachers, ask about the extent of their training in yoga's eight limbs: *yamas* (how to treat others), *niyamas* (how to treat yourself), *asana* (postures), *pranayama* (breath control), *pratyahara* (withdrawal of the senses), *dharana* (focused concentration), *dhyana* (meditation), and *samadhi* (oneness with all beings). The teacher you choose should be well versed in all eight limbs, along with texts such as the Bhagavad Gita, the Yoga Sutras of Patanjali, *Ramayana*, Yoga Upanishads, and *The Hatha Yoga Pradipika.* Although there are many more wonderful books, these provide a good foundation for yogic philosophy.

The teacher you engage should be comfortable wearing and working with a lavalier microphone and cueing up music through the church's sound system or through a Bluetooth speaker. They should also have experience with helping create a sacred aesthetic, augmenting the church worship space with things like candles, soft lighting, incense, fabric, green plants, or flowers. Their ability to hold space for students should come naturally through characteristic traits of kindness, compassion, empathy, love, and respect. The yoga teacher needs to be welcoming, open-minded, and able to change the planned asana flow to match the age and ability level of the students. Unlike a studio class, which tends to draw the same students of similar ability week after week, workshops draw participants of varying abilities, so the teacher must be on the lookout for those who appear to be struggling and make instant adjustments. Sirena manages to help everyone feel welcome, including those participants who are able to do nothing more than lie down on a pew in their street clothes and listen.

The teacher should have experience in offering options for the postures, using props such as yoga blocks, blankets, and straps. The more supported the students feel, the more likely they are to return to a future workshop. If they felt the asana practice was too difficult or they were embarrassed by not being able to complete the full expression of a pose, they might be discouraged from participating again. The teacher should be adept at using welcoming and accessible language to build confidence in students. Keep in mind that not all students have their own props such as mats, blocks, blankets, or straps, so plan to have extra on hand.

When searching for a teacher, don't overlook those in the parish who may be certified and experienced yoga teachers. Also consider asking the yoga practitioners in the parish to recommend teachers whose gentle manner and knowledge of yogic philosophy they most admire. If there's no obvious candidate, advertise for applicants. The community bulletin boards at local studios can be good places to post a flier describing what you're looking for. Remember, you don't need a teacher who can teach advanced arm balances and lead students through vigorous, sweat-inducing flows. You are looking for someone with a solid spiritual grounding, an intellectual curiosity, and an open and compassionate heart.

What is important is that the teacher have a familiarity with and respect for Christianity. Sirena was raised Catholic but isn't presently a member of any church. Her passion for sharing the intersection of yoga and Christianity arose through building a close relationship with me in the Monday night bike shop yoga classes. Sirena has a deep admiration for Christian history, texts, and ritual, and we each found a willing and open discussion partner in each other. Inviting a teacher in with no faith background or respect for Christianity may invite challenges. Remember, he or she will be working alongside clergy and will be teaching vestry members, parishioners, and community members. Sirena has built wonderful relationships with many parishioners and attends church services on occasion, which has blossomed into sharing the spirit of God and community.

Physical Space, Music, and Hospitable Setting

A sacred physical space can create a sense of home within. Home is where we live and is also within us, a place for which we often find ourselves yearning. There is an inner sense of home within all of us, and during our lives the way and the degree to which we experience this varies. Yoga in the Church is a wonderful opportunity to help your students feel deeply connected to God and the flow of life. The physical space you create for your participants is vitally important to their sense of going home within.

We chose to teach these workshops *in the church*. We guided participants to set their mats on the floor in the nave in front of the pews, down the center aisle, the transept aisle, on the chancel between the choir pews, and even in front of the altar. In warmer weather (and during the pandemic) we held workshops on the church lawn and patio. By being in the worship space and by employing things like incense, candles, and sacred music, we wanted to affirm that yoga is an act of worship and appropriate for a sacred space. We wanted to make it easy for participants to find this same sacred space within themselves.

When setting up the space, do so with attention to both safety and inclusivity. Because St. John's is a downtown church in a city of over 100,000 people, and because our workshops tend to be in the evenings, we chose to lock the church doors once the last attendee had arrived. The open floor space in our church is limited, so we required attendees to sign up in advance. That way we ensured we did not have more participants than available floor space for mats. We created a guest list and checked people off at a welcome table as they arrived and paid. We call people by name as often as we can to create a heart connection with them and to help them feel like they belong in the space. If you can manage to enlist a parishioner to staff the welcome table, all the better. Be sure that access to restrooms is clearly signed and that water is available for participants. St. John's campus is big, so we take care to use outdoor signage to point people to the correct building and doors. Don't assume your attendees have experience walking into a church or feel comfortable doing so. Simple signs such as "YOGA THIS WAY →," "YOGA IN HERE," and "WELCOME TO YOGA IN THE CHURCH" can go a long way toward creating a hospitable experience for your participants from the moment they set foot on the church campus.

An important safety consideration is the use of candles. As lovely as burning candles may be, take care to place them well away from participant mats and traffic flow. One option is to leave them unlit until all participants are in place on their mats and then to light them as part of the opening ritual or meditation. We use both real candles and faux, battery-operated ones, choosing the latter where a stray leg or arm might accidentally make contact. A spray bottle of water, close at hand, can address any accidents. It's also worth noticing the airflow in the church. For our first workshop we set up a centrally located table with artfully arranged tapers. It was lovely, but what we failed to account for was that we had chosen a spot that's a virtual wind tunnel in our worship space. At the end of the workshop, we realized to our dismay that the candles had burned wildly, spewing wax everywhere like a child's science fair volcano. We did not make that mistake again.

For those with a sensitivity to perfumes, scented candles or incense can be an irritant. If you plan to burn incense, state that in your advertising. Burn it well away from the area where participants will be practicing, or extinguish it before the session begins. Before a workshop starts, decide on lighting, and designate who will dim the lights at the appropriate time. Have small flashlights or booklights available so you can read your notes in low light. Check that microphones have fresh batteries and sound systems are set at an acceptable level. If you are using your phone to play music, make sure to turn off notifications so it does not ring or vibrate during the workshop. That can be very distracting as well as embarrassing.

We have music playing as people arrive and during the asana flows. We also use it to support a meditative Savasana. We do not play music during our spoken teachings, to minimize background noise and help participants focus on what we are saying.

Participants need to sign a waiver (at least one time), so have it available when they check in. A waiver is a requirement of the yoga teacher's insurance policy and is also a layer of protection for the church. Participants can pay in advance through your church's online donation system, an independent system like PayPal or Venmo, or as they arrive for the workshop. At the conclusion of the workshop have pens available for participants to complete surveys, if you use them. Participant feedback is invaluable.

If we have a handout or small gift relating to the workshop topic, we pass it out afterward so as to not be a distraction during class. We offer a lot of philosophical and theological content during a workshop, and putting some of it in a handout releases the note-takers from having to jot down what we say and allows them to relax and listen. We regard handouts as value-added pieces that allow participants to take home some of our teachings and reflect on them in the days to come. If we create a handout, we take care to include citations for the source material we use. Sometimes a workshop topic inspires us to send participants home with a small gift. In the workshop on community ("The Journey Is Better Together"), Sirena told of an ancient Chinese belief that an invisible red thread connects those whom we are destined to meet. She and her daughters made red string bracelets with a heart bead and placed it on the wrists of the participants. As they wore it, it served as a lovely reminder of the teachings of community and to be mindful that we are all connected.

Even the smallest and most mundane details contribute to creating sacred space. Joseph Campbell said, "Your sacred space is where you can find yourself again and again."[11] We hope Yoga in the Church participants can find that interior sacred space within during our workshops, and can realize they carry it with

11. Joseph Campbell, *Reflections on the Art of Living: A Joseph Campbell Companion* (New York: Harper Perennial, 1995), 180.

them always so they can return to it at will. Creating a unique workshop experience where participants feel fully at home with others and within themselves is a blessing they can hold in their hearts until they return next time.

Building the Ministry from the Ground Up

Just as an asana is properly "built" from the ground up, so is a new ministry of Yoga in the Church. In Boulder, Colorado, yoga is extremely popular, so the pushback we experienced from church members was relatively minor. The same may not be so in your community. Patience and sensitivity in building up this ministry are key.

We started slowly with a handful of yoga classes and play-shops in the parish hall during Lent. Despite promoting these opportunities to parishioners, participation was sparse. It was only when we moved into the worship space, committed to exploring and teaching the philosophical and theological intersections, and opened the workshops to the community that the ministry began to flourish. Even in our yoga-saturated community, we found a surprising number of attendees were beginners. If you find that most of your attendees are unfamiliar with yoga, don't expect to launch into Yoga in the Church. Start with basic instruction in the church's parish hall or a large open classroom. Invite the curious to a free or low-cost play-shop. This can be a chance for students to learn the names of the postures, proper alignment, and how to modify a pose to accommodate their body's particular needs. During a play-shop, talking, questions, and interruptions are encouraged. Once students understand how to safely attain some basic asanas, you can begin to move your ministry into the worship space and introduce silence, guided meditations, and philosophical and theological teachings.

Social media can be wildly effective or a burden, depending on how much time you have to invest. We established a Facebook Group for Yoga in the Church and create advertisements to post in our timeline about upcoming events. We share details about workshops and offer links so people can easily sign up. Ideally, you'll find a parish volunteer who is interested in maintaining the page.

Email campaigns can also be quite effective. We started our email list with the few people who showed up for the beginner classes and play-shops. We found a couple of extremely excited evangelists, who shared news of our first workshop with great numbers of their friends outside the church. This was a real gift to us. Sirena also advertised in her regular in-studio yoga classes, her community drop-in classes, and on her own social media. As a result, many people asked to join the mailing list. Our Meetup group generated interest but also yielded a lot of folks who signed up and then were no-shows. We use an email system through Mail Chimp, which houses contact information and tags and provides unique template opportunities for pictures and links. Using an email system can help you track who opens the emails and how often. Understanding your audience is key. Your outreach will evolve, shift, and grow as you understand which marketing campaign is most effective.

Your community will grow as you provide opportunities to come together and share in teachings, yoga, and discussions. We always allow time for visiting before the workshops begins. If the workshop is small, build in introductions and invite participants to share why they decided to attend. Yoga has a distinct way of creating a feeling of connection to oneself, after which one realizes the overwhelming sense of connection to others and to God. These realizations are the building blocks of community. B. K. S. Iyengar said, "Yoga is firstly for individual growth, but through individual growth, society and community develop."[12]

Pandemics and Other Disasters

One year into our Yoga in the Church offerings, the Covid-19 pandemic started, and as we write this book, it is still going on. We had to shift gears immediately, just like everyone else in the world, and figure out how to offer our workshops online. We decided to use the Zoom platform and used the church's donation site for payment. The day prior to a workshop, we sent out a welcome email to registrants and encouraged them to set up their own sacred space in their home. We suggested they light candles or incense, brew a hot drink, and place a journal and pen next to their mat. Sirena thought through which props might be needed and got creative, suggesting the use of a large book instead of a block or a rolled blanket instead of a bolster. She suggested having a blanket and pillow available for Savasana. Giving participants specific information about how to create a sacred and comfortable space helped them feel prepared and in control at a time when much in life was well beyond our control. Sirena's compassionate heart understood that some people struggle to practice yoga through a computer screen, so she assured participants that sitting, listening,

---

12. B.K.S. Iyengar, "B.K.S. Iyengar Quotes and Sayings—Page 3," Inspiring Quotes, 2021, *https://www.inspiringquotes.us/author/5461-b-k-s-iyengar/page:3.*

and being in virtual community with others was perfectly acceptable. In the midst of the isolation forced on us by the pandemic, some people just wanted to feel connected to others.

As a parent obliged to move her children to online school, Sirena witnessed their struggles to stay engaged with a computer screen. Given this, she made the wise suggestion to trim our two-hour workshops. We still offered time for welcome and opening check-ins and for questions and discussion following the workshop. It was important to us to be able to offer the same welcoming and safe space as we did in the church. Like many group activities that have gone from in-person to online during the pandemic, attendance at Yoga in the Church Online has declined somewhat. We acknowledge this without alarm and look forward to a time when the church can once again be safely filled with practitioners.

5

A YEAR'S WORTH OF YOGA-IN-THE-CHURCH WORKSHOPS

> Don't be afraid to adapt new ingredients into your own techniques, and traditional ingredients into new recipes.
>
> *–Jose Garces, Ecuadorian American chef and restaurateur*[1]

AS WE DISCUSSED OUR VISION FOR THIS BOOK, Sirena and I were clear that we wanted to give you a template or basic recipe for a Yoga in the Church workshop and more ingredients than you need so you can make each workshop your own—and can even create multiple workshops on the same topic. I also trust our material will inspire you to add relevant stories, quotations, bits of scripture, and theology that have special meaning for you.

The Basic Recipe

Each workshop will follow this same format. We'll offer far more components than you need or should use in a single workshop. It's like the advice I was given in seminary when we were learning how to preach: don't put every good idea you've ever had about God in a single sermon. Often, less is more.

Workshop focus. We developed concise titles for each workshop that are informative and ear-catching. We suggest times of the year, church seasons, or seasons in a human life when each workshop might be especially appropriate.

Music suggestions. Music choices abound. We offer you what we have used and found to be powerful and moving. A blend of yoga music and Christian music is appropriate. Simple and repetitive music such as Taizé songs can support a flow. Don't compete with yourself by trying to teach a complex bit of theology or philosophy with music playing in the background. Do engage soft

1. "Recipe Quotes," BrainyQuote, accessed October 21, 2021, *https://www.brainyquote.com/topics/recipes-quotes.*

music to accompany an opening or closing meditation. If you are fortunate enough to have a live musician, work with them to create pieces that support the teachings, flows, or meditations. Whether recorded or live, music is there to support the workshop and should not be overbearing.

Pranayama. Sometimes we offer pranayama, sometimes a guided meditation, and sometimes both. We assume your yoga teacher has a basic understanding of pranayama techniques through his or her teacher training and practice. If you'd like a brush-up or additional ideas, we like the book *Pranayama: A Path to Healing and Freedom*.[2]

Teachings from yogic philosophy (yoga teachings). What do the yoga sutras have to say about the topic? What do other Vedantic texts have to say? This is where your yoga teacher will probably have ideas and resources of their own to contribute.

Teachings from Christian scripture and theology (Christian teachings). What scripture stories or verses amplify the points made by the yogic philosophical texts you've cited? What bits of theology (or science) do likewise? We choose yogic and Christian texts that each affirm what the other is saying, but from time to time we do offer contrasts—for example, "The yoga sutras say such and such, but Christian scripture has something a bit different to say." This honors our intent not to throw both traditions in the wash and make them come out the same color.

Each Christian teaching is identified by a ✝, and each teaching from yogic philosophy is identified by a lotus flower icon. It's up to you to customize your workshop. After you assemble it, we urge you to read through what you've chosen and ensure there is a logical flow from one teaching to the next.

Suggested asana flows. We have designed these flows to reflect the mood or theme of the workshop. Your teacher may wish to substitute different asanas or create a flow of their own. We offer these flows so you have a ready-made workshop if you don't have the time or inclination to design a flow.

Closing meditation. This optional component can be a pre-Savasana meditation or can occur during it. If a spoken meditation is offered, it's designed to let participants integrate the theme of the workshop quietly and without movement.

2. Allison Gemmel LaFramboise with Yoganand Michael Carroll, *Pranayama: A Path to Healing and Freedom* (Seattle: CreateSpace, 2015).

Extras. This is where we pose postworkshop discussion questions for those who like to hang around and chat. We might suggest handouts or small take-home gifts (see chapter 4). This is optional, but these little extras can set your workshops apart from all the other yoga workshops out there, and that's good when you're starting out and trying to build a community of practitioners.

When scheduling, we usually opt for early evening so people with 9-to-5 jobs can easily attend. When we planned our first Yoga in the Church workshops, we wanted to be sure that both young adult singles and parents could participate, so for this target audience, evening was a must. We also stuck with a weeknight, betting that young families would be off skiing or playing on the weekend. The demographics of the community beyond your church doors will help inform what time is best. If you're in a place popular with retirees, an afternoon class may be preferable. Give some thought to a day and time, and try to stick with your choice for all your workshops. If people know you're always offering yoga on a Tuesday at 4:00 p.m., it's one less detail they have to remember. If your church is like mine, once you find a free day and time in the church calendar, you claim it and guard it jealously.

Because our nave simply doesn't have enough open floor space to accommodate all the people who want to attend, we've tried offering the same workshop on two consecutive nights or two consecutive weeks. From the perspective of teacher stamina, we found the latter to be easier.

In this chapter, we offer these workshops in no particular order and suggest you consider what's happening in the world around you and choose from them accordingly. In creating and scheduling these, we discussed what was happening on the national and international stages and also closer to home on the Front Range of Colorado. This is not to suggest you must seek out a pressing societal concern or a natural disaster and schedule a Yoga in the Church workshop in response to it. Just be aware that such things tend to motivate people to seek out sanctuary, where they can rediscover purpose and meaning, rest in the grace of some benevolent power beyond themselves—which we Christians call God—and recalibrate. In addition to responding to current events, we considered how our topic did or did not correspond to the liturgical season in the church calendar. We considered the humble rhythms of human life, like back-to-school time, summer vacations, graduations, and other thresholds of accomplishment, as well as days of observance like Earth Day. We also took note of happenings in the cosmos, like solstices and eclipses. By syncing our workshops with what was happening in the world around us, we hoped to make them more relevant.

You may wish to take a different approach and instead target particular audiences, like single people, the bereaved, cancer survivors, teens, or chronically overscheduled working adults.

In our workshops, sometimes we begin with yogic teachings and sometimes with Christian teachings. Just be sure that the overall flow of teaching forms a coherent dialogue between the two traditions.

When we began offering workshops, each one ran close to two hours in length and included a short discussion session following. We had so much we wanted to share with people and weren't as disciplined as we could've been about holding ourselves to a timetable. As part of each workshop, we also asked participants to complete a short survey. (You can find the survey we used at the end of this chapter.) It was the feedback received on those surveys that encouraged us to trim the workshop length from two hours to one. We still may exceed that one hour slightly, but overall, we're accomplishing our goal of respecting people's time. Or, as an old maxim advises, we always leave them wanting more.

From my training as a preacher, I know I speak about 150 words per minute when I am preaching or teaching. When Sirena and I are creating a workshop, we use this as a way to measure how long it will take to present what we have written. When we began developing workshops, we started with fewer teachings of longer duration, but now tend to favor more teachings of shorter duration. Bear in mind the processing capacity of your listeners. Our brains process information much faster if we are reading it than they do if we are hearing it. In other words, slow down.

In yoga teacher training one learns the art of welcoming participants. Your yoga teacher should be experienced in doing that and in creating a warm and hospitable environment where questions are welcome, imperfection is celebrated, and everyone is encouraged to be the steward of their own body and experience. What we added, which is important, was language to reassure people we're not out to convert anyone, nor are we trying to show the superiority of one tradition over the other. In my welcome I said, "The more I do yoga the more I see beautiful intersections between yogic philosophy and Christian theology. Tonight is a chance to explore those intersections in an intentional way." On other occasions I offered, "We'll look at what the yoga sutras and Christian theology have to say on the topic of _____. Our intent is not to yoga-ize Christianity nor to Christian-ize yoga, but rather to notice and appreciate those places where they overlap." I also acknowledged the rightness of being in my parish's historic worship space: "I'm honored to welcome you into a worship space where, for more than one hundred years, people have come to pour out their souls to the divine and to seek union with the divine. I believe these walls are therefore saturated with prayer, so I invite you to let the holy residue of those prayers hold you and guide you through tonight's practice." However you say it, the welcome portion of a Yoga in the Church workshop is a time to answer the unasked question that will be on the minds of many of your participants: Do I really belong here? That answer, of course, is yes!

Workshop 1: The Yoga of Surrender

Workshop Focus: This workshop explores the idea of the surrender of the self (the ego) to God. It is particularly suited to the season of Lent or Holy Week (especially Good Friday), when Christians are already considering what it means to surrender and to practice the way of Jesus who surrendered his will, his agenda, his earthly attachments, and finally his very life to God. This workshop could also be appropriate in the aftermath of a natural disaster or a crisis time in national (or personal) life, when something larger than oneself has wrested control of life.

Music Suggestions:

Peter Gabriel, "With This Love," track 16 on *Passion: Music for the Last Temptation of Christ,* Real World Studios, 1989. (arrival and check in)

Jean Rausis, "[Aramaic] Psalm 53 in Georgia (for Pope Francis)—Remastered," YouTube video, 5:06, October 5, 2016, *https://www.youtube.com/watch?v=Xq3UX8yIBZI* (opening meditation and flow).

Angelika, "Abwoon," track 2 on *Benediction*, 2009, *https://angelikahealingmusic.com/music/* (closing Savasana).

Pranayama: Sit comfortably, and switch legs if you like. Inhale arms up, exhale hands down to the sides (two times), then inhale arms up, exhale hands into dhyana mudra (empty bowl mudra)—left hand is on bottom, right hand is on top, and connect the tips of your thumbs. We empty out in order to allow what will come. Deep inhale through the nose, exhale through the mouth (three times). Arrive.

Close your eyes, and connect with your soft, natural breath. Let go of your day, your week, your expectations, and arrive on your mat. Reflect on your intentions for coming tonight. What moved you to make the decision to join us? What sparked your curiosity? Your interest? Let go of your expectations for tonight, and allow the path to unfold as it should, knowing whatever comes up tonight is exactly what you need. Let's lie down on our backs in Savasana.

Christian Teachings:

✟ The word *surrender* can conjure up edgy feelings in us, especially when it's used in conjunction with religion or spirituality. We're right to feel edgy because *surrender* is a military word. It means

- to cease resistance to an enemy or opponent and submit to their authority;
- to yield to the power, control, or possession of another upon compulsion or demand; or
- to give (oneself) over to something (such as an influence).

Surrender is a military word and not a spiritual one, and yet it's been used widely in the language of Christianity. This is unfortunate because it suggests that God is the enemy or opponent, the One who demands power and control over us. In fact, nothing could be further from the truth.

If you struggle with this image of God, consider this story: One day in seminary Susan translated the Psalm 23 from the ancient Greek. It's such a popular psalm, but she had always disliked it because of the line that reads: "He [God] makes me lie down in green pastures." Whenever she heard that line she could not help but bristle and wonder, "What if I don't *want* to lie down?"

As she translated, something marvelous happened: she could not find in her lexicons the Greek word for "makes lie down." She looked and looked. She checked several reference books. Finally, it occurred to her to pull the Greek word apart to see if she could translate the component pieces into English. That sort of worked, and when she reassembled the word and wrote out the English translation of the verse, here's what she got:

> The Lord is the shepherd of me. I shall want for nothing. He sings the earth to me [or sings the ground or soil to me].

What a different message this sends about God. The Holy One is not the enemy or the opponent demanding we lie down—demanding power over us. Rather, the Holy One is a lover, calling to us to surrender into the divine arms so we can be held. This new way of understanding profoundly changed Susan's faith and her spiritual life and made it possible for her to let go, to give herself over to the divine.

✝ The etymology of the word *surrender* reveals that one of its roots is "rendre,"[3] meaning "to give back." If we can think of ourselves as coming from God and our lives as a journey back home toward God, we might think of "surrender" as giving ourselves back to the One from whom we came.

This does not mean it is easy or without pain. In the Bible, all four Gospels—Matthew, Mark, Luke, and John—all tell the story of Jesus's arrest by Roman soldiers in the Garden of Gethsemane. Even though Jesus went away peacefully with the military authority, the word *surrender* is not used by any of the four Gospel writers.

One thing that *does* occur in all four accounts is Jesus asking the Father, "Please, if it is possible, let me not have to do this. Let me not have to be arrested, betrayed, mocked, tortured, and killed." And even as he uttered those words he understood that all these things were part of his calling.

This [Holy Week] is the week in the Christian tradition when we remember a period of hours in the life of Jesus. Those hours were not meant to show us a God who demands the death of his son in payment of some debt we have created by being sinful and disobedient. Rather, they were meant to show us that God's very nature is self-giving. As the human incarnation of God, Jesus *chooses* to give himself over to the military authorities, for divine love knows no enemies.

There's a parallel story in Buddhism, from the Chinese invasion of Tibet in the mid-twentieth century. A soldier entered a monastery and thrust his rifle into the belly of a meditating monk. The monk kept meditating. The soldier was taken aback by this and said to the monk, "You don't understand: I have the power to take your life." The monk briefly opened his eyes, smiled at the soldier, and replied, "No, it's *you* who doesn't understand. I have the power to *let* you."[4]

That's the nature of pure love—it gives unconditionally of itself. We can attempt to betray, mock, and destroy love, but a few days from now, on Easter, we'll be reminded that love is impossible to kill. Love is greater even than death.

✝ Part of surrender is letting go of attitudes that do not serve us. Using anger as an example, writer Cynthia Bourgeault reminds us that if it seems too difficult to let go of a strong emotion or desire, we can console ourselves with the knowledge that for now we are only practicing. She says, "Remember that letting go [of your anger] is only for this moment. [You are not making] a blanket

3. Online Etymology Dictionary, s.v. "surrender," accessed October 21, 2021, *https://www.etymonline.com/word/surrender*.

4. Bourgeault, *The Wisdom Jesus*, 181.

vow never to be angry again; [you are merely releasing your anger] in the present moment. Anger will almost certainly be back. But each time you are able to pass [that anger] through the light-beam of your compassionate attention, it loses more and more of its hold on your being."[5]

The attitudes that do not serve us usually arise from the cravings of our false self. Those cravings or desires can be grouped into three energy centers, three unhealthy motors that drive much of our behavior: We might crave or desire safety and security, and loathe change. We might crave or desire affection and esteem, and seek approval from others. We might desire power and control, and engineer ways we can have it.

When any of these desires claim us and direct our behavior, we become their slave. Surrender is the spiritual practice of releasing those desires that seek to enslave us. Cynthia Bourgeault offers a litany of release:

> I let go of my desire for security and survival.
> I let go of my desire for esteem and affection.
> I let go of my desire for power and control.
> I let go of my desire to change the situation.[6]

Yoga Teachings:

In the yoga sutras, the idea of surrender revolves around the niyama *Ishvara Pranidhana*. A niyama is one of the eight limbs of yoga and is the action of spiritual observance. *Ishvara* stands for God, and it is understood that God is formless yet also taking the form of everything. God is whatever you personally define God to be. *Pranidhana* is defined as the action of turning on, directing toward, and surrendering to. This surrender to God, the Universe, or a higher being shifts our perspective from "I" and the "ego" to the "source" of our "true Self." It provides a pathway through the obstacles of our ego toward our own divine nature—toward grace, peace, love, and freedom. We each have our own personal relationship with the divine, and that relationship can serve as our own personal yoga practice.

Ishvara Pranidhana takes time to cultivate. It takes time to slow down, become more mindful of our breath, our actions, our reactions. It takes time to build a trust and shift our perspective, letting go of our ego to commune with God, the Universe, a higher being. As our inner sense of direction grows,

5. Ibid, 180.

6. Ibid.

it increasingly guides our thoughts, speech, and actions. We cultivate a deeper inner listening, set daily intentions, pray, or meditate. As Shiva Rea, a modern yogini, said, "Ishvara pranidhana could be called 'heartfulness' practice; it awakens our constant devotion to the Source of life and keeps our hearts open to the Divine in every moment, no matter what arises."[7] It is in letting go that transformation happens.

Suggested Asana Flows: In the yoga sutras, we call "letting go" *aparigraha*. It is the practice of nonattachment to things, people, outcomes, yoga poses, self-images—to name a few. Think of something you are holding onto in this moment, at this time in your life. Bring to mind whatever you know you need and want to release and let go of. Whatever you've chosen, bring it close to your heart in this moment.

Stanza 1: Start the vinyasa flow; have participants repeat to themselves on the right-side warrior III:

> I let go of my desire for security and survival.
> I let go of my desire for esteem and affection.

Stanza 2: Continue the vinyasa flow on left side; have participants repeat to themselves on the left-side warrior III:

> I let go of my desire for power and control.
> I let go of my desire to change the situation.

Stanza 3: When in child's pose in the asana flow, have participants repeat:

> I surrender.

Warm-up

- Mountain pose
- Hands over head pose
- Anjali mudra at heart center
- Hands over head pose
- Forward fold—halfway lift—forward fold
- Plank

7. Shiva Rea, "How to Practice Ishvara Pranidhana—A Practice of Surrender," *Yoga Journal*, August 28, 2007, *https://www.yogajournal.com/yoga-101/philosophy/the-practice-of-surrender/*.

- Baby cobra
- Downward-facing dog
- Tabletop
- Cat-cow

Flow

- Downward-facing dog
- Crescent high lunge right leg forward
- Crescent high lunge, with arms lifted, then cactus arms, arms lifted, then airplane arms, bend at waist, arms lifted
- Warrior III, balance on right leg (offer arm options: airplane, heart center, pointing forward); repeat stanza 1 from option #3 above
- Forward fold—halfway lift—forward fold
- Plank
- Baby cobra
- Downward-facing dog
- Crescent high lunge left leg forward
- Crescent high lunge with arms lifted, then cactus arms, arms lifted, then airplane arms, bend at waist, arms lifted
- Warrior III, balance on left leg (offer arms options; airplane, heart center, pointing forward); repeat stanza 1
- Forward fold—halfway lift—forward fold
- Plank
- Baby cobra
- Downward-facing dog
- Child's pose; repeat stanza 3

Cooldown

- Tabletop
- Bird dog, right arm forward and left leg back; then switch sides
- Cat-cow
- Lie on back and squeeze legs into belly
- Supine twist, both sides
- Savasana

Closing Meditation: We suggest no music during the closing meditation. Invite participants into Savasana, guiding them to settle in and quiet their minds, and to repeat to themselves:

> I surrender to what is and to what will be.
> I surrender to trust in myself and my path,
> To trust in God, as I understand God to be;
> I surrender to pure compassion and boundless love.

Play the singing bowl to initiate the end of Savasana. Move participants to a seated position, with hands at heart center in anjali mudra (prayer position). Offer gratitude to the participants for coming together.

Extras: Consider giving each participant a smooth stone and, using permanent makers, taking a moment after the workshop for each person to write on the stone what they wish to surrender. Discuss how they might release that weight—for example, burying the stone or dropping it into a body of water.

Workshop 2: Just Breathe–What Yoga and Christianity Have to Say about Anxiety

Workshop Focus: This workshop offers tools one can use to lessen anxiety. People respond with anxiety to the national mood; political divisiveness, racial injustices, a pandemic, global unrest or war, impacts of climate change, and the widening wealth gap set a baseline of anxiety. Threshold moments in a human life (job changes, new school, relationship or family changes, health scares) often add a layer of anxiety atop the baseline.

Everyone experiences anxiety. When we're anxious it's normal to hold our breath. This means we reduce our intake of oxygen at a time when we need it most. Come and learn techniques to release anxiety and reawaken the ability to breathe in a way that will calm and recenter you.

We included guided journaling as part of this workshop. If you choose to do that, be sure to include that in your advertising so people can bring their own journals if they wish. Also have pens and paper on hand for those who don't bring their own. If your ministry budget permits, giving participants a small blank book as part of this workshop and suggesting they bring it to future classes can be a gracious way to let participants know you hope they will return.

Music Suggestions:

Peter Gabriel, "With This Love," track 16 on *Passion: Music for the Last Temptation of Christ*, Real World Studios, 1989. (arrival and check in)

Alex Dav, "Relaxing Hang Drum Music," YouTube video, 6:00:19, July 26, 2020, *https://www.youtube.com/watch?v=gv0m2OW0s7o*. (opening meditation and flow)

Simon Lockyer, "Drifting Away," track 1 on *Antenatal Relaxation*, Angelworks, 2007. (closing Savasana)

Pranayama: We offer you two options for an opening pranayama.

Option 1: In yoga, *pratyahara* means the withdrawal or transcendence of the senses. This limb of yoga recognizes that the mind tends to go toward whatever stimulates the senses, and responds with pratyahara, the practice of drawing the senses inward, relieving them of their external distractions. Pratyahara forms a bridge between the externally focused limbs of yoga, such as asanas, and the internally focused ones, such as pranayama. The yoga sutras explain this, bridging from pranayama to pratyahara:

> The fourth kind of pranayama takes us beyond the domain of inner and outer.
> Then the light of the intellect is unveiled.
> And the mind is prepared for steadiness.
> The senses retire from their objects by following the natural inward movement of the mind.
> From this comes supreme mastery of the senses.[8]

This short meditation will be the first step as you become aware of your senses and internal and external distractions. Find a comfortable seat, close your eyes, and find your natural breath. Rest your hands on your thighs or knees.

Here we are, [*day and time*]. We are here with community in a sacred and safe space. As we reflect on the day, take note of the challenges and stress that may have left you with anxiety. Take a deep breath in through the nose; open the mouth and exhale (two more times). However your week is going, bring your awareness to your body and your presence on your mat tonight. With eyes closed and inhaling through the nose, start at the crown of your head and lengthen your spine. Lift the crown of your head toward the sky. Now lift your

8. *The Yoga Sutras of Patanjali*, trans. and introduced by Alistair Shearer (New York: Bell Tower, 1982), II:51–55, 111–12.

rib cage, taking care to keep your shoulders relaxed. Open your mouth and exhale, feeling a heaviness descend into your hips, legs, and feet. Feel your connection to the mat, the floor, the ground.

Bring your hands to your belly. Inhaling, feel your belly rise, and then on an exhale feel your belly fall. Let this subtle movement be a reminder of your physical body and connection to your breath. Our senses collect and react to everything around us. Let's engage them to help ground us:

> What do you hear? [*Pause after each question.*]
> What do you smell?
> What do you see, without seeing?
> What do you taste, without eating?
> What do you feel physically?
> What do you feel emotionally?
> What do you feel spiritually? [*Offer a longer pause here.*]

As we begin tonight's practice, I offer an evening meditation adapted from the writings of the sixteenth-century Christian mystic, Teresa of Avila:

> Let nothing, O Lord, disturb the silence of this night.
> And here in the gathering darkness let me relax in your presence.
> There is nothing to be afraid of.
> There is everything to hope for.
> I may not become perfect overnight, or be instantly blessed . . .
> But little by little I will grow in knowledge of the road that leads to heaven.[9]

I invite you to consider that heaven is not a destination but a state of mind. [*Observe a moment of silence.*]

Find your breath. Let go of your week. Let go of your expectations. Take tonight what resonates most with you; leave what doesn't.

> Just breathe.
> Flutter open the eyes.
> Let's move our bodies. [*Move from here into an asana flow.*]

Option 2: There's a saying that worrying about tomorrow steals the strength and joy of today. In yoga, we talk a lot about being in the moment. Anxiety

9. Teresa of Avila, *Let Nothing Disturb You*, ed. John Kirvan (Notre Dame, IN: Ave Maria Press, 2008), 18.

steals that moment away from us. Do you know what else anxiety steals from us? Our breath.

In Sanskrit, the word for a person's soul, the real Self of an individual, is *Atman*. In German, the word for "to breathe" is *atmen*. Across cultures, there seems to be an understanding that breath and soul are connected and are the source of life. We breathe unconsciously all the time. A practice in yoga called *pranayama* raises our awareness of the breath and teaches us to *consciously* breathe.

Pranayama cleanses and detoxifies the body and clears the mind. Leading yoga teacher and author Mark Stephens says, "As we breathe, so we feel, and in breathing more freely and fully, we feel more freely and fully."[10] Pranayama gives us the power to change how we feel and shows us that we can find bliss in the present moment simply by consciously focusing on the breath. Pranayama can corral our runaway-horse thinking and gently ground us in the present moment.

The basic awareness breath allows you to build an initial foundation for your pranayama practice. Everyone's natural breath varies, depending on their physical, emotional, mental, and spiritual condition. Breath can be compromised by depression, anxiety, respiratory conditions, and distractions. Becoming attuned to your natural breath is a process of learning what you are doing that restricts its emergence.

Lie down on your back, inhaling through the nose and exhaling through the mouth at your own pace. Let your hands or fingers lay on your belly to bring even more awareness to the filling and emptying of breath.

Inhaling—What does it feel like? Where do you feel the breath enter and then settle? Where is the movement of the breath? Does it get stuck somewhere along the way?

Exhaling—Where do you first feel the movement of the exhalation? Does the breath rush out? Are you pushing it out? What changes do you feel in your body or fluctuations in your mind upon the exhale?

The basic awareness breath has a balancing influence on the entire cardiorespiratory system. It releases feelings of irritation and frustration and helps calm the mind and body. Other benefits you might experience include an increased amount of oxygen in the blood; relief of tension; the sense of a freer flow of *prana* (the vital energy or life-force that moves through the body

---

10. Mark Stephens, *Teaching Yoga: Essential Foundations and Techniques* (Berkeley, CA: North Atlantic Books, 2010), 239.

as we breathe); regulation of blood pressure; and increased feelings of presence, self-awareness, and meditative qualities.[11]

Yoga Teachings:

A tool that can also be used in conjunction with pranayama is *dharana*, which is focused concentration. There are several types of dharana—walking meditation, watching a candle flicker, listening to the breath (Ujjayi), or even listening to a song on repeat. One of my favorite methods of dharana is mantra. Deepak Chopra describes mantras as "mind transportation": *man-* (mind) and *tra* (transportation).[12] Our minds are always switched on, always thinking. The Buddhists call this the "monkey mind." The question for us is, How do we tame it? One way is to give the mind a mantra, something to concentrate on, focusing only on that one thing so we can detach from everything else around us.

You may already be familiar with some Sanskrit mantras such as "Om" or "Om Shanti." Mantras can also be used in English. Think of a word or phrase that resonates with you deeply. Examples might be, "Peace in me" or "All is well." Mantra is similar to a prayer repeated over and over. The Jesus Prayer long used in Christianity is one such example: "Lord Jesus Christ, have mercy on me, a sinner." Another is, "Be still, and know that I am God." Some Christians engage the breath, inhaling on the first portion of the prayer and exhaling on the second. It's possible to engage a pranayama technique in this same way if you wish.

In yoga, a mantra is repeated audibly, then silently, then mentally without words. This orderly process of repetition is called *japa*. The yoga sutras teach the practitioner how to use japa and a mantra (in this case "Om") to clear the mind:

> The Lord is a unique being who exists beyond all suffering.
> Unblemished by action, He is free from both its cause and its effects.
> In Him lies the finest seed of all knowledge.
> Being beyond time, He is the Teacher of even the most ancient tradition of teachers.
> He is expressed through the sound of the sacred syllable *OM*.
> It should be repeated and its essence realized.

11. Melissa Eisler, "Learn the Ujjayi Breath, and Ancient Yogic Breathing Technique," Chopra, January 29, 2016, *https://chopra.com/articles/learn-the-ujjayi-breath-an-ancient-yogic-breathing-technique.*

12. Tris Thorp, "What Is a Mantra?," Chopra, January 14, 2021, *https://chopra.com/articles/what-is-a-mantra.*

> Then the mind will turn inward and the obstacles that stand in the way of progress will disappear.[13]

Repeating a mantra may be done at any time and is especially helpful before bed. I repeat the same mantra 108 times and find it helps pull me away from my worries and provides me with a meditative vibration to lull me to sleep. I've also used it when I have been anxious: during pregnancy or before a big meeting at work. Mantras are excellent for beginning meditators because they offer a tangible focus.

Let's practice. Come to lie on your back as we did when learning the pranayama. As you start the basic awareness breath, or ocean waves, breath, think about a small phrase that brings you calm and peace. Use this mantra to send an anchor down into the ground of your being. Let it gently hold your mind still and in place.

Christian Teachings:

✝ Anxiety arises when we tell ourselves we are alone and that alone we must face what frightens us. But this is not true. There is a divine being, a divine energy, a divine love that surrounds us and is available to us always. God knows the hairs of our heads, knows when a sparrow falls from a tree, knows our thoughts before they leave our lips,[14] and loves *all* aspects of us—even those we consider unlovable. God neither slumbers nor sleeps and is with us always. We are not alone.

Anxiety arises when we allow ourselves to dwell in the future. Indeed, anxiety has been called the present anticipation of future pain. This kind of future dwelling is different than planning and dreaming, which are good. Planning and dreaming are positive future thinking. Anxiety is negative future thinking and does not serve us.

If we choose to partner with the God who awaits us, then we learn to allow the future to unfold one day at a time. We respect that pace and do not hurry into tomorrow. There is a divine rhythm to the universe, and sometimes it is slower than we feel we must move. Instead of shoving and pushing into tomorrow, we can learn to allow ourselves to be led there by the author of peace. The peace of God, which is so abundant it's beyond understanding, starts to fill our hearts and minds. We can learn to meet each new day with curiosity instead of dread.

---

13. *The Yoga Sutras of Patanjali*, I:24–29, 94.

14. Luke 12:7; Matt. 10:30; Matt. 10:29; Ps. 139:2–4; Ps. 121:3–4; Matt. 28:20.

✝ Father Thomas Keating was a monk recognized as a founder of the practice of Centering Prayer. One of Keating's teachings was about the False Self. A person's False Self is comprised of three energy centers. Each of these three emerges in early childhood, as our little vulnerable selves attempt to deal with experiences of fear or depravation. The three energy centers are safety and security, affection and esteem, and power and control. It is not wrong to need these things. Where we run into trouble, says Keating, is when these needs become so exaggerated that the need itself drives our behavior.[15]

Our logical minds would acknowledge that we don't have the ability to manage our environment. Our logical minds would acknowledge that of course there will be times in life when we don't feel safe or secure, when we don't feel affection or esteem, when we don't feel powerful or in control. If our needs are in check or in balance, we are able to listen to our logical selves. But when our needs become so exaggerated they step in and drive us, those needs make us anxious because we cannot possibly meet them.

Buddhists call this *grasping* or *clinging* and caution that it is a prescription for misery. Christian scripture calls this a failure to live in the present. Each one of us had different childhoods, so each one of us tends to have different needs that always seek to jump in the driver's seat.

As you work to understand the root of your anxiety, it's helpful to understand which of these energy centers is usually the most active in you. When you are feeling anxious, invite yourself to hit "pause" and ask yourself the question, "What need do I have right now that isn't being met? Could that need be so exaggerated that it is driving my behavior? Can I release at least some of this need and hang onto only what seems logical?"

Take your journal or piece of paper. I'll pose two reflection questions and invite you to take two minutes to respond to each. I'll let you know when the first two minutes has passed.

The first journaling prompt: Reflect on the first decade of your life through the lens of the three energy centers: safety and security, affection and esteem, power and control. Did any of these feel chronically lacking in your childhood home? Does one more than the others stand out as usually lacking?

---

15. Thomas Keating, *Invitation to Love: The Way of Christian Contemplation* (New York: Continuum Publishing, 2001), 5–13; Lowell Grisham, "The Three Energy Centers of the False Self," Episcopal Café, September 12, 2011, *https://www.episcopalcafe.com/the_three_energy_centers_of_the_false_self/*.

The second journaling prompt: Think about the anxiety you feel today as an adult. Can you link that anxiety to one or more of the three energy centers (safety and security, affection and esteem, power and control)?

✝ Many antidotes exist for anxiety, among them moving your body, eating a healthy diet, getting adequate sleep, nurturing supportive relationships, and seeking the help of a therapist when it feels like other strategies aren't working. One antidote may surprise you. It is portable and free. It is the practice of gratitude.

Researchers have found a causal link between sustained and high anxiety and increased inflammation in the body. High levels of inflammation in the body can weaken our immune system and increase our risk for physical illness. Chronic worry causes wear and tear inside our bodies.[16] Because there is a physical cost to being anxious all the time, it behooves us to find ways to reduce or even eliminate our anxiety.

Enter the practice of gratitude. Researchers have looked at what happens when people spend as little as five minutes a day engaged in the practice of gratitude journaling. They found this practice, over a two-month period, lowered stress and improved sleep. A gratitude journaling practice lowered the markers in the blood for inflammation, including the hemoglobin A1C, which is "associated with risk of heart failure, heart attacks, diabetes, chronic kidney disease, various cancers, and death."[17]

If you are curious to learn more about the science of gratitude, check out the work of Dr. Robert Emmons, a professor of psychology at the University of California, Davis.[18] He's written or contributed to a number of books about gratitude, and they are listed on his faculty webpage. He's also conducting an interesting study about gratitude and God.

Thinking about the physiological benefits of gratitude has helped me read certain scripture in a new way. I want to share two. The first (verse 24 from Psalm 118) is probably familiar to you: "This is the day that the LORD has made; let us rejoice and be glad in it." The second is from the first letter to the Thessalonians (5:18): "Give thanks in all circumstances; for this is the will of

16. Melville, "Worry, Anxiety Tied to Increased Inflammation"; Vogelzangs et al., "Anxiety Disorders and Inflammation in a Large Adult Cohort," e249; Felger, "Imaging the Role of Inflammation in Mood and Anxiety-Related Disorders," 533–58.

17. Smith et al., *The Gratitude Project*, 44.

18. "Robert Emmons," UCDavis, accessed October 21, 2021, *https://psychology.ucdavis.edu/people/raemmons*; Jane Hart, "Practicing Gratitude Linked to Better Health: A Discussion with Robert Emmons, PhD," *Alternative and Complementary Therapies* 19, no. 6 (2013): 323–25, *https://www.liebertpub.com/doi/abs/10.1089/act.2013.19609?journalCode=act*.

God in Christ Jesus for you." I've always read these as directives, as commands: Be grateful, because if you aren't, God will be offended. Give thanks because if you don't, God will be disappointed.

But what if instead, these scriptures are a prescription for our mental and physical health? Rejoice and be glad in this day, and you'll be doing your body and brain a favor. Give thanks in all circumstances because it'll help your body and brain stay healthy, and health is what God wills and wishes for you. Pretty different, yes?

Take your journal or piece of paper. I'll offer a short meditation and invite you to take three minutes to respond. I'll let you know when the time is drawing to a close.

Meditation: Think back on this day, this one day. Take yourself through each part of the day, beginning with your waking up in bed. What felt good about it? Take yourself through your morning routine of bathing, eating, praying, feeding pets or children. What did you cherish? Walk with yourself into the day as it unfolded—into work or errands or social time or physical activity. What went well? What stands out in your memory as pleasurable? Now bring yourself from the height of your day to this moment. For what are you grateful right now? Think about the remainder of the evening ahead. To what do you look forward?

Journaling Prompt: As you consider this one day, for what are you grateful? What people? What conversations? What learning? What experiences? Smells? Tastes? Sounds? Tactile sensations? Emotions? Journal about as many as you can in the next three minutes. Don't worry about writing sentences. Just respond with words and phrases.

Allow three to four minutes for journaling before checking back in.

Now look at what you have written. Witness the vast and varied riches of gratitude buried beneath the surface of this one day. No matter what is happening in the world, look at all the ways you have been blessed.

✝ In the Gospel of John (20:19–22) the friends of Jesus are hiding in a locked room, fearful that the same people who crucified Jesus are now coming for them. Suddenly, Jesus himself appears in their midst and says, "Peace be with you!" He shows them his wounds of crucifixion to prove who he is. Again, he says, "Peace be with you!" and then he breathes on them and says, "Receive the Holy Spirit." In ancient Greek, the word for "Spirit" can also mean "breath" or "wind." So, you can think of Jesus inviting his friends to receive the holy breath.

If we can conceive that God is in all things, then God inhabits even the air we breathe. Each time we inhale, we take in something of God. And each time we exhale, we return something of God to God. With this understanding, every breath is holy. Christian teacher Richard Rohr says that our "simple breathing models [our] entire vocation as human being[s]. [We, like Christ, are incarnations] of matter and spirit operating as one."[19] Be comforted, then, that when you draw in air, you draw in the substance and peace of God.

You also inhale some wisdom. Many scientists believe that every breath we take is connected to those who came before us. They tell us at least a few particles of the air we inhale are part of the exhalations of people all the way back to Julius Caesar—perhaps even earlier. Every single breath we take has been associated with another living organism before we draw it in. When you are feeling anxious and unequipped to deal with life, gently remind yourself that you are breathing in some of the wisdom of the ancients.[20]

Suggested Asana Flows:

Warm-up

- Child's pose
- Tabletop
- Cat-cow
- Downward-facing dog
- Forward fold—halfway lift—forward fold
- Hands over head pose
- Twist right, left hand in front, right hand behind
- Hands over head pose
- Twist left, right hand in front, left hand behind
- Hands over head pose
- Forward fold
- Plank
- Puppy pose
- Sphinx pose
- Downward-facing dog
- Child's pose

19. Richard Rohr, *The Universal Christ* (New York: Convergent Books, 2019), 99.

20. Sam Kean, *Caesar's Last Breath* (New York: Back Bay Books, 2017), 10–11.

Flow

- ➢ Child's pose
- ➢ Downward-facing dog
- ➢ Right leg forward
- ➢ Warrior I
- ➢ Warrior II
- ➢ Reverse warrior with bound lower arm
- ➢ Extended side angle
- ➢ Triangle
- ➢ Five-pointed star (quarter turn to the left)
- ➢ Wide-legged fold
- ➢ Goddess pose—close eyes, lift heels
- ➢ Five-pointed star
- ➢ Wide-legged fold
- ➢ Runner's lunge, left side
- ➢ Lift hips, walk hands to top of mat, repeat runner's lunge, right side
- ➢ Plank
- ➢ Puppy pose
- ➢ Sphinx pose
- ➢ Child's pose
- ➢ Repeat opposite side

Cooldown

- ➢ Seated, soles of feet touching, knees out; fold
- ➢ Sage pose, right knee bent, twist left
- ➢ Sage pose, left knee bent, twist right
- ➢ Boat pose
- ➢ Lie on back and squeeze legs into belly
- ➢ Supine twist, both sides
- ➢ Savasana

Closing Meditation: Play a singing bowl (or other gentle signal) to initiate the end of Savasana. Bring participants to a seated position, with hands at heart center in anjali mudra (prayer position). Offer one of these closing prayers:

Option 1: Instead of fighting against feeling anxious, Father Keating suggests we look at our anxiety, welcome it, feel it, and then release it. By doing this we're not seeking to indulge our anxiety. We're not trying to justify or amplify it. We're simply acknowledging it.

By welcoming our anxiety, we're not inviting it to move in and live with us. Instead, we're acknowledging the reality of it so it ceases to have authority over us. We're pulling it out of the dark into the light so we can see it for what it is: one feeling among many feelings that a human being experiences. Once we welcome it, it's time to let it go—to release it—for it is not serving us.

> Welcome, welcome, welcome.
> I welcome everything that comes to me today
> because I know it's for my healing.
> I welcome all thoughts, feelings, emotions, persons,
> situations, and conditions.
> I let go of my desire for power and control.
> I let go of my desire for affection, esteem,
> approval and pleasure.
> I let go of my desire for survival and security.
> I let go of my desire to change any situation,
> condition, person or myself.
> I open to the love and presence of God and
> God's action within. Amen.[21]

Option 2: This closing prayer is adapted from a prayer of the sixteenth-century Christian mystic, Teresa of Avila:

> Let nothing, O Lord, disturb the silence of this night.
> Let nothing make me afraid.
> Rather, as darkness descends and this day ends,
> Let me retreat to the very center of my being, my soul,
> Which you . . . have created in your own image and likeness
> And which you have chosen as your home.
> Make me aware of your presence and of my likeness to you.
> Let us speak together in the silence of the night . . .
> [And] let me find . . . [peace] in your presence.[22]

---

21. Tom Frontier, "The Welcoming Prayer by Father Thomas Keating," My Shepherd King, January 13, 2018, *https://www.myshepherdking.com/the-welcoming-prayer-by-father-thomas-keating/*.

22. Teresa of Avila, *Let Nothing Disturb You*, 18.

Extras: Consider offering participants the use of eye pillows. If you are handy with a sewing machine, you might create eye pillows filled with dried lavender. Consider offering fresh-brewed chamomile or other calming tea. If teaching the use of mantras, try offering small pieces of heavy, fine-quality paper (such as watercolor paper) on which participants can write mantras. Using a hole punch and some ribbon allows participants to tie their mantras someplace visible at home.

Workshop 3: The Journey Is Better Together: What Yoga and Christianity Have to Say about Community

Workshop Focus: This workshop explores the importance of community to a healthy human life. It is a natural for September, when families who've scattered for summer vacations are returning to school and Sunday worship. Sunday school, paused perhaps for the summer months, starts up and children and their parents reconnect. Church ministries of fellowship and study resume in full swing. In the world beyond the church, fall marks a time when people return from summer travels and look more to the company of others. Homecoming events at high schools and colleges are ways of celebrating the importance of the community that is built when people share life together for four years.

Music Suggestions:

Peter Gabriel, "With This Love," track 16 on *Passion: Music for the Last Temptation of Christ*, Real World Studios, 1989. (arrival and check in)

Mahanta Das, "Reiki Mahamantra," *Reiki Mahamantra*, Evolution Music, 2017. (opening meditation and flow)

Bombay Dub Orchestra, "The Greater Silence," track 6 on *Bombay Dub Orchestra*, Six Degrees Travel Series, 2017. (closing Savasana)

Pranayama: *Simhasana* (lion's breath) stretches the muscles of the face, relieves tension, and begins to build some inner heat to prepare the body for asanas. With its exaggerated facial expression and stuck-out tongue, it's also a delightful icebreaker, especially if participants can face one another.

Yoga Teachings:

Of the many definitions of yoga, one of the most loved is "union." Yoga is the union of Self, body, mind, and spirit. Yoga is also the union between the self, nature, the cosmos, and other humans. The communities in which we live and thrive are dense networks of relationship and union. The yoga sutras, considered the "bible" of yoga, also represent union. The word *suture* means to sew or mend together a wound. *Suture* is derived from the Sanskrit word *sutra*, which means to thread or weave together an understanding of direct and indirect experiences as encountered by the Self and by the Self among others. It is a sacred thread that connects us all.

In this workshop we come together to weave a connection and create community. Our aim is to see union in the world around us and within us. The practice of yoga is about a relationship we have with ourselves. What does your relationship with your Self look like? How do you treat your Self? With love? Compassion? Patience? In the yoga sutras, Patanjali tells us that we need to have these qualities in relationship to our Self. Then, of course, we can think of all these things in relationship to others.[23]

The word *community* can be defined as a group of people who live in the same area, as a unified body of individuals with common characteristics and interests.[24] In yoga, a group of like-minded people gathered to support each other—to share meals, friendships, and resources—is called a *sangha*. *Sangha* is a Sanskrit word meaning association, assembly, company, and community. The famous Vietnamese monk Thich Nhat Hanh described sangha as a "beloved community that includes people who are engaged in serving and bringing joy to one another and [who] inspire each other to contribute."[25] Hanh stresses the contribution of every individual to the community and of the community to the greater world. This contribution that you bring to your community is considered your dharma.

Dharma is the act of duty or service you are providing within your life and community in this very moment in time. Your dharma may change over time as it flows through the ever-changing life experiences. What is your dharma within your community, and how has it changed over time?

Yoga sutra 2.24 (*tasya hetuh avidya*) is translated as, "Obviously, all this is due to the ignorance of the spiritual truth or oneness." Ignorance alone is the cause for polarization, the fictitious separation that is the sole cause for the desire to become aware of "another" and for the contact of "the other."[26]

---

23. Carolyn Gregoire, "Yoga Philosophy 101: Take Yoga Off the Matt and into Your Relationships," *Yoga Journal*, September 27, 2016, *https://www.yogajournal.com/lifestyle/take-yoga-mat-relationships*.

24. *https://www.merriam-webster.com/dictionary/community*.

25. Jen Mergler, "Sangha," Yoga Parkside, August 2, 2021, *https://www.yogaparkside.org/sangha/*.

26. Swami Venkatesananda, "Enlightened Living: A New Interpretative Translation of the Yoga Sutras of Maharsi Patanjali," The Chiltern Yoga Trust, 2008, 21.

In American culture, individualism has been prized and prioritized. This idea of being unique or special can either set us apart or help us fit into a particular community. We are social creatures, but our egos, unchecked, can separate and polarize us and cause us loneliness. There is a term in yoga called *avidya*, which is a Sanskrit word for "misconception and ignorance." It implies thinking that you exist alone and not as a part of a larger whole. Avidya leads us to give undue value to our individualism and to our independence from the larger collective. In truth, though, we are never separate from the community, except in our minds. A practice of yoga can help us quiet the chatter and know the universal truth of connectedness.

Through our practice we come to realize that we are not only individual in mind but also a part of the community. We are not that different and separate from it, but we are of it, contributing our dharma, our service, our duty. To think otherwise is *avidya*, ignorance.

A practice of yoga can help us learn that in caring for our individual needs, we care for the whole community. And when we reach out and care for what's around us, we heal ourselves as well.

Christian Teachings:

✝ A progressive Christian theologian named Richard Rohr has suggested that the basic template of reality is Trinitarian; in other words, it's relational.[27] God is not a one-man or one-woman deity. The nature of God is relationship. If you read the creation story in the first chapter of the book of Genesis, the words are clear: "Let *us* make humankind in *our* image, according to *our* likeness." (v. 26 emphasis mine). Whoever or whatever God is, this implies that God is not an autonomous character acting in isolation. Rather, God is—at least in part—relationship.

We're made to be relational creatures, and we are most ourselves when we're in community. Each one of us has something unique and precious to offer a community. You might think of the human body with all its parts, each having a unique role to play but each in close relationship with all the other parts. Paul, in Romans 12:4–5 NIV, described Christian community in that same way: "For just as each of us has one body with many members, and these members do not all have the same function, so in Christ we, though many, form one body, and each member belongs to all the others."

---

27. Richard Rohr, keynote address, May 8, 2018, Episcopal Diocese of Colorado Annual Clergy Conference, May 8, 2018.

Recent findings in brain science agree with what progressive Christianity is saying:

> fMRI research shows that [in our brains] there are two distinct networks that support social and non-social thinking and that as one network increases its activity the other tends to quiet down—kind of like a neural seesaw. Here's the really fascinating thing. Whenever we finish doing some kind of non-social thinking, the network for social thinking comes back on like a reflex—almost instantly.
>
> Why would the brain be set up to do this? We have recently found that this reflex prepares us to walk into the next moment of our lives focused on the minds behind the actions that we see from others. Evolution has placed a bet that the best thing for our brain to do in any spare moment is to get ready to see the world socially. I think that makes a major statement about the extent to which we are built to be social creatures.[28]

✠ Community is where we learn to teach, where we learn to learn, where we learn what it means to be a friend to someone, where we learn what it means to bear someone's burden with them—to be in solidarity with them in their pain, or grief, or suffering. Community is where we learn the impact of our words and actions—especially when those words and actions are not well chosen—and community is where we learn to forgive and to be forgiven. Community is a school for learning how to better love.

Community attracts the divine spirit—Jesus told his friends that when two or three of them gathered in his name he would be in the midst of them. I think that's a way of saying that loving, generous relationships attract divine energy. Community attracts divine energy. If God is—at least in part—loving relationship, then like attracts like.

Richard Rohr says, "Living in community means living in such a way that others can access me and influence my life and that I can get 'out of myself' and serve the lives of others. Community is a world where brotherliness and sisterliness are possible."[29] Rohr goes on to describe community as a network of caring, cooperative relationships. It is the antidote to a society that seems to run on individuality, greed, and competition.

---

28. Gareth Cook, "Why We Are Wired to Connect," Scientific American, October 22, 2013, *https://www.scientificamerican.com/article/why-we-are-wired-to-connect/*.

29. Richard Rohr, "Church Was Supposed to Be an Alternative Society," Center for Action and Contemplation, May 9, 2018, *https://cac.org/church-was-supposed-to-be-an-alternative-society-2018-05-09/*.

✝ Author David Brooks says our nation has experienced a fundamental shift over the last half-century. Prior to the 1960s the group or community was the fundamental unit of American society. Today, it is the individual that is the fundamental unit. Our culture has become one of hyperindividualism, and the previous network of bonds between people has slowly been weakening.[30] In the last forty years alone, the number of Americans who report feeling lonely has doubled.[31] People of faith believe that the divine is guiding us back toward community. Richard Rohr says that "God will always bring yet more life and wholeness out of seeming chaos and death. It seems to be the very job description—and full-time occupation—of God. [People of faith] hope for a different future, a transition to a society less destructive, more peaceful and more whole."[32] People of faith spend their lives living in a way that helps to midwife that transition.

Rohr also says, "As Dr. Martin Luther King Jr. saw clearly in the last years of his life, we face a real choice between chaos and community—we need a moral revolution. If that was true fifty years ago, then we must be clear today: America needs a moral revival to bring about beloved community."[33] When we come to understand how connected we already are—that what we do to others or do to the earth we in fact do also to ourselves—then we are doing our part to bring about this revival, this transition to beloved community.

Protestant pastor and political leader Rev. Dr. William Barber writes, "The main obstacle to beloved community continues to be the fear that people in power have used for generations to divide and conquer God's children who are, whatever our differences, all in the same boat."[34] Richard Rohr adds that "it takes a contemplative, nondual mind to see foundational oneness—that we truly are 'in the same boat.'"[35]

Rohr says,

---

30. David Brooks, *The Second Mountain: The Quest for a Moral Life* (New York: Random House, 2019), 10.

31. Michael Hendrix, "Hyper Individualism and Radical Diversity Are Leaving Americans Very Lonely," *Dallas Morning News*, April 21, 2018, *https://www.manhattan-institute.org/html/hyper-individualism-and-radical-diversity-are-leaving-americans-very-lonely-11164.html.*

32. Rohr, "Church Was Supposed to Be an Alternative Society."

33. Richard Rohr, "The Beloved Community," Center for Action and Contemplation, May 8, 2018, *https://cac.org/the-beloved-community-2018–05–08/.*

34. Rohr, "The Beloved Community."

35. Rohr, "The Beloved Community."

> The goal of the spiritual journey is to discover and move toward connectedness and relationship on ever new levels, while also honoring diversity. We may begin by making connections with family and friends, with nature and animals, and then grow into deeper connectedness with those outside our immediate circle, especially people of races, religions, economic classes, gender, and sexual orientation that are different from our own. Finally, we can and will experience this full connectedness as union with God. For some it starts the other way around: they experience union with God—and then find it easy to unite with everything else.
>
> Without connectedness and communion, we don't exist fully as our truest selves. Becoming who we really are is a matter of learning how to become more and more deeply connected. No one can possibly go to heaven alone—or it would not be heaven.[36]

✝ In South Africa, the word *ubuntu* describes a sacred sense of community. The word came into use in the mid-nineteenth century and was popularized in the 1950s. *Ubuntu* means "I am, because of you."

Desmond Tutu said of *ubuntu*: "Ubuntu is very difficult to render into a Western language. It speaks of the very essence of being human. [If you have *ubuntu* you are] generous, hospitable, friendly, and caring and compassionate. You share what you have. It is to say, 'My humanity is inextricably bound up in yours.' We belong in a bundle of life."[37] I like the image of community as a bundle of life in which my humanity is inextricably bound up in yours. Tutu continues, "A person with *ubuntu* is open and available to others, affirming of others, does not feel threatened that others are able and good, for he or she has a proper self-assurance that comes from knowing that he or she belongs in a greater whole and is diminished when others are humiliated or diminished, when others are tortured or oppressed."[38]

These words of Desmond Tutu describe an ideal for life in community. When we provide a safe space for one another, when we encourage one another, when we find space to collaborate, we create community. Better yet—*ubuntu*.

---

36. Rohr, "The Beloved Community."

37. Kate Torgovnick May, "I Am, Because of You: Further Reading on Ubuntu," TEDBlog, December 9, 2013, *https://blog.ted.com/further-reading-on-ubuntu/*.

38. "Community Quotes," Goodreads, accessed October 21, 2021, *https://www.goodreads.com/quotes/tag/community*.

Suggested Asana Flows:

Warm-up

- Child's pose
- Tabletop
- Thread the needle—both sides
- Cat-cow
- Flip toes under, hips to heels, tops of feet to floor, hips to heels
- Tabletop
- Extend right leg out, press toes into mat for right calf stretch; switch legs
- Downward-facing dog
- Forward fold—halfway lift—forward fold
- Hands over head pose
- Goddess the arms, hands up, arms down to goddess (do this a few times)
- Forward fold—halfway lift—forward fold
- Plank
- Child's pose

Flow

- Mountain pose
- Chair pose
- Step left foot back into high crescent lunge
- Warrior I
- Exhale to bend at waist, and airplane arms behind
- Warrior I
- Warrior II
- Reverse warrior
- Turn left into five-pointed star
- Wide-legged forward fold; walk hands to right foot
- Standing splits, balancing on right foot
- Step left foot up to the right at the top of the mat into forward fold
- Hands over head pose
- Goddess arms
- Hands over head pose

- Side bend right, send bend left
- Forward fold
- Plank
- Lower down onto belly
- Baby cobra
- Downward-facing dog
- Forward fold
- Repeat opposite side

Cooldown

- Lie on belly for sphinx pose
- Bow pose
- Flip to back
- Fish pose
- Figure 4 right ankle on top of left knee; lift left foot as option to go deeper into hip
- Figure 4 left ankle on top of right knee; lift right foot as option to go deeper into hip
- Butterfly pose on back, soles of the feet together
- Supine twist, both sides
- Savasana

Closing Meditation: Before Savasana, pass out red thread bracelets. Ours featured a heart bead and were adjustable. Play the singing bowl to initiate the end of Savasana. Bring participants to a seated position with hands at heart center in anjali mudra (prayer position).

There is a Chinese belief that an invisible red thread connects those who are destined to meet. You came to this workshop for a reason. This red thread tied around your wrist is a reminder that who you are and what you contribute to the community around you is important.

Extras: At the close of the workshop, a designated photographer can snap a few smartphone photos of the in-the-moment community that the workshop attendees have created. Because you have everyone's email address when they registered for the class, these photos can be easily shared. Doing so by email gives you an opportunity to thank people for coming and to invite them to create community with you again in a future class.

Workshop 4: Let It Be–Forgiveness and Compassion in Yoga and Christianity

Workshop Focus: We were created to live lightly, freely, and joyfully, yet many of us only visit these states instead of living in them. The struggle to forgive—ourselves as well as others—entraps and weighs us down. Developing the ability to have compassion for self and for others is a key to living more of our lives in the territory of joy.

This workshop could be offered in preparation for family holiday gatherings. Who among us has not dreaded them from time to time, especially in these days of deep division in our nation? It might also be interesting to offer this workshop in the fall, at the time of the Jewish holy day of atonement, Yom Kippur. Some congregations might want to make this yoga workshop part of a healing weekend that includes a liturgy of reconciliation or healing, with an opportunity for the laying on of hands and praying.

We have witnessed tears in some of our Yoga in the Church workshops, and this topic more than others is likely to bring up excruciatingly painful feelings in some people. Have a plan for how you intend to support those participants who are struggling emotionally. A bowl of cool, damp cloths; a person trained in pastoral listening (a clergyperson, lay minister, or therapist) and a private space apart from the class; abundant tissues; lavender or herbal-scented pillows; prayer shawls; a companion with whom to walk a labyrinth—these are just a few possibilities for how to care for those whose tears ask for our compassion.

Music Suggestions:

Peter Gabriel, "With This Love," track 16 on *Passion: Music for the Last Temptation of Christ*, Real World Studios, 1989. (arrival and check in)

Brigitte Lesne and Discantus, *Hildegard von Bingen Hortus Deliciarum*, Alliance, 2006. (opening meditation and flow)

Dead Can Dance, "Devorzhum," track 8 on *Spiritchaser*, 4AD/Warner Bros. Records, 1996. (closing Savasana)

Pranayama: Guide participants through the Ujjayi breath.

Yoga teachings:

Keys are indispensable items. They give us access to our cars and offices. They provide a layer of protection for things we value. They guard the sanctuary of our homes. According to the yoga sutras, there are also keys we can use to unlock our heart. These keys help us overcome distractions, face challenges, and cultivate kindness for others and for ourselves. Using these keys grants us access to our compassionate and forgiving heart.

Yoga sutra 1.33 says to be friendly toward and rejoice with those who are happy. Perhaps a spouse or friend gets an unexpected but much deserved promotion at work. They cannot wait to share their good news with you. Perhaps your initial reaction is envy. After all, you have worked hard too. No one has ever recognized *you* with a promotion or a raise. This reaction comes from the ego, not from the heart. Patanjali says, "By that jealousy, you will not disturb other people, but you disturb your own serenity."[39]

The Sutra continues by telling us to cultivate compassion for the less fortunate and unhappy. You may or may not know the source of someone else's unhappiness, but by expanding your awareness you may recall a time you, too, were suffering. Perhaps a young mother is struggling. You recall your own struggles and sense of isolation from being home alone all day with young children. Your empathy leads you to offer help. Even a small gesture of kindness can be a lifeline for someone.

The next part of the Sutra tells us to honor the virtuous. Being virtuous is not limited to saintly folk like Buddha, Jesus, Ghandi, or Mother Teresa. Even ordinary people possess noble qualities. Nischala Joy Devi says, "Everyone has human limitations along with her or his greatness; it is up to us to choose which aspects to focus on."[40] When we see the best in others, we will be inclined to see the best in ourselves. When we see the worst in others, we inevitably find the worst in ourselves. Think for a moment of some of the people you encountered today. Can you find beautiful and noble qualities in them?

The Sutra concludes by telling us to disregard toward the wicked. It sounds easy in theory, but we know it can be hard in practice. Family members, coworkers, even friends all rile us up from time to time. Joy Devi explains this portion of the sutra by saying, "Equanimity to those whose actions oppose your values."[41] To have or show equanimity means to maintain calmness, mental composure, and an evenness of temper. It is empowering to know we can make the choice not to engage. Recall the words of Martin Luther King Jr., who said, "The ultimate measure of a person is not where they stand in

39. Sri Swami Satchiidananda, *The Yoga Sutras of Patanjali* (Buckingham, VA: Integral Yoga Publications, 2012), 52.

40. Nischala Joy Devi, *The Secret Power of Yoga* New York: Three Rivers Press, 2007), 82.

41. Devi, *The Secret Power of Yoga*, 83.

moments of comfort and convenience, but where they stand in times of challenge and controversy."[42]

The way we treat others is often how we treat ourselves. You not only can use these keys on others but also yourself. These keys offer you a door to peace of mind.

Yoga sutra 1.8 reads, "Misunderstanding comes when perception is unclear or tinted."[43] Sometimes misunderstandings lead to grudges. Sometimes grudges can be nursed for so long they are carried to the grave, leaving a legacy of trauma and hurt to the next generation. Most of us have had the unhappy experience of a small misunderstanding ballooning into a major conflict. Perception is a highly personal thing: your perception may be quite different from another's. Asking for clarification and then listening quietly can help bring things into better focus.

There is often fear around forgiveness, that we are letting the offender off the hook. However, by holding hatred in our hearts, we are only causing suffering in ourselves. We are binding and entrapping ourselves in a web of frustration, anger, and grief. To forgive is to loosen the cords and to clear the way to freedom. Forgiveness is ultimately a stepping-stone to compassion for yourself and others. Joy Devi says, "As the heart softens through forgiveness, the understanding emerges that they are also hurt and unhappy, and then forgiveness melts into compassion."[44]

In yogic philosophy, the author of forgiveness is not God but one's own self. Because there is no doctrine of sin, there is no corresponding doctrine of divine judgment. To find forgiveness, the yoga practitioner studies the Yoga Sutras in order to better learn about the self and find ways to change behavior. Part of this learning is to reflect on those who cause us frustration and suffering and to study our reactions to their behavior. Misunderstandings are seen as opportunities for learning. The Yoga Sutras provide guidance and support for making more virtuous decisions.

Yoga sutra 2.33 states, "When presented [with] disquieting thoughts or feelings, cultivate an opposite, elevated attitude. This is called pratipaksa bhavana."[45] As challenging as this is to put into practice, it is intended to help the practitioner change their mind about a troublesome person or situation, rather

42. Devi, *The Secret Power of Yoga*, 84.

43. Devi, *The Secret Power of Yoga*, 31.

44. Devi, *The Secret Power of Yoga*, 84.

45. Devi, *The Secret Power of Yoga*, 172.

than trying to change the behavior of the troublesome person or the nature of the situation. It hands control to the practitioner, reminding us that we alone are in control of our own thoughts and feelings. We can acknowledge them and then can make the decision to move on from them to something better.

Christian Teachings:

✝ (If using this teaching, be sure to preface it with the teaching on the four keys of the Yoga Sutras.) Christian scripture has an interesting parallel with the Yoga Sutra's four keys: in the Gospel of Matthew (16:19), Jesus speaks to his disciple Peter and says, "I will give you the keys of the kingdom of heaven, and whatever you bind on earth will be bound in heaven, and whatever you loose on earth will be loosed in heaven."

In the ancient world the giving of keys symbolized the granting of authority. The ancient rabbis believed that God held four keys in his hand, and those keys unlocked rain, the ability to conceive, resuscitation of the dead, and the growth of crops.[46] Modern readers of this verse tend to interpret the keys more like the Yoga Sutras—in other words, the keys to the kingdom of heaven are attitudes and practices that help us let go of the things that trouble our tranquility and inhibit our ability to love.

We believe that the kingdom of heaven or the kingdom of God is not limited to some realm located beyond the edge of our galaxy. Heaven is also among us and within us. Jesus himself says as much in the Gospel of Luke (17:20–21 KJV), when he states, "For behold, the kingdom of God is within you."

Given that, you could say that whatever hurts and misunderstandings we "bind" or dwell on will take up residence in our heart, mind, and spirit and swirl around in there incessantly. Whatever we can't release becomes a weight we carry with us, and it hampers our ability to live in a state of tranquility—to live in the kingdom of heaven. Conversely, whatever hurts and misunderstandings we can "loose," or let go of, cease to take up space in us, and they cease to have such power over us. We are thus free to live in a mind and soul state of heaven.

✝ Forgiving others is impossible to do until we can grasp that God has forgiven us. We cannot extend to others mercy and forgiveness if we have not already experienced them ourselves. Most of us struggle on occasion to accept that we have deep intrinsic value and are beloved in God's sight. But learning to accept our own beloved-ness as well as our fallibility is important if we are to

46. "Power of the Keys," Bible Gateway, accessed October 21, 2021, *https://www.biblegateway.com/resources/encyclopedia-of-the-bible/Power-Keys.*

be able to forgive and love others. Consider yourself as an L-shaped piece of pipe. Forgiveness from God flows continually down into you and then in turn flows out from you to others. This is what the Lord's Prayer is getting at in the line, "Forgive us our trespasses, as we forgive those who trespass against us." If we refuse to forgive someone, it blocks the pipe, and a blocked pipe prevents us from receiving forgiveness from God. In other words, it's in our best interest to forgive others, in order to keep the channel clear and open.

"To forgive," says Richard Rohr, "is not to forget. [To forgive is a] letting go [that] frees up a great amount of soul-energy [and] liberates a level of life you didn't know existed. [To forgive] leads you to your True Self."[47] Forgiving others is important to our own spiritual growth, and spiritual growth is a life-long process in which we learn to peel back the layers of our False Selves and see ourselves for who and what we truly are.

Rohr says that when we mature spiritually we

> become aware that we are not the persona (mask) we have been presenting to others. . . . Facing [this] reality is . . . liberating because we recognize that our manufactured self-image is nothing substantial or lasting; it is just created out of our own mind, desire, and choice—and everyone else's opinions of us! We must become intentional about recognizing and embracing our shadows. Religion's word for this is quite simply forgiveness, which is pivotal and central on the path of transformation.[48]

✝ We tend to make God's forgiveness a lot more conditional and convoluted than it really is. Jesus had a way of seeing into someone's heart. If he sensed someone felt wretched about what they had done, he pronounced them forgiven. In the Gospel of Luke (7:44–50), Jesus was at a dinner party when in walked a woman we might describe as an award-winning sinner. She went over to Jesus, didn't say a word, and lovingly anointed his feet with ointment. She cried on his feet and tenderly dried them with her hair. The other guests protested, but Jesus stopped them and said, "her sins, which are many, are forgiven—for she loved much. But he who is forgiven little, loves little" (Luke 7:47, ESV).

In the centuries after his death, the followers of Jesus made forgiveness a lot more complicated. As Christianity became institutionalized, forgiveness was only granted after confession, penance, and indulgences. Sins got categorized

---

47. Richard Rohr, "Forgiveness: Weekly Summary," Center for Action and Contemplation, September 2, 2017, *https://cac.org/forgiveness-weekly-summary-2017-09-02/*.

48. Richard Rohr, "Facing Reality," Center for Action and Contemplation, September 13, 2019, *https://cac.org/facing-reality-2019-09-13/*.

into venial and mortal sins—less serious and more serious. The more serious the sin, the more complicated the process of forgiveness.

We need people like William Langland to set us straight. Langland lived in England in the fourteenth century. Not much is known about him, but we do know that he was somewhat against organized religion. Perhaps he didn't have much use for the church that had made granting forgiveness such a complex process. In defiance, he wrote, "The worst sin that man may think or do is to the mercy of God no more than a live coal thrown into the sea."[49] Think about that for a moment: the most horrific thing you could possibly do has no more effect on God or God's adoration of you than a burning charcoal briquette has on the cool, fathomless expanse of ocean. Psst. Gone. Done. Rendered as nothing. It's like a mosquito trying to bite the face of the moon. Remember that, and perhaps then it will be easier for you to accept that you are beloved.

Suggested Asana Flows:

Warm-up

- ➢ Easy seat
- ➢ Head rolls: right ear to right shoulder, left ear to left shoulder, both directions
- ➢ Seated side bend right; seated side bend left
- ➢ Seated twist right; seated twist left
- ➢ Lie on back and hold knees into chest, rocking left to right
- ➢ Extend left leg straight, bend right knee into chest, and hold right foot for half happy baby; switch sides
- ➢ Bridge pose
- ➢ Lie on back and hold knees into chest, rocking front to back
- ➢ Table top
- ➢ Cat-cow
- ➢ Downward-facing dog
- ➢ Forward fold—halfway lift—forward fold
- ➢ Hands over the head pose
- ➢ Mountain pose
- ➢ Be seated

49. Wikipedia, s.v. "William Langland," last modified July 15, 2021, *https://en.wikipedia.org/wiki/William_Langland*; Wikipedia, s.v. "*Piers Plowman*," last modified October 20, 2021, *https://en.wikipedia.org/wiki/Piers_Plowman*.

Flow

- ➢ Table top
- ➢ Downward-facing dog
- ➢ Lift right leg for three-legged downward dog
- ➢ Warrior I, right leg forward
- ➢ Warrior II
- ➢ Extended side angle
- ➢ Triangle
- ➢ Turn left into five-pointed star
- ➢ Wide-legged fold
- ➢ Runner's lunge, left knee bent
- ➢ Wide-legged fold
- ➢ Walk hands to front right foot
- ➢ Step left foot up to right foot; forward fold
- ➢ Chair pose
- ➢ Eagle arms
- ➢ Eagle legs—option for balance
- ➢ Hands over head pose
- ➢ Forward fold
- ➢ Plank
- ➢ Lower down onto belly
- ➢ Baby cobra
- ➢ Downward-facing dog
- ➢ Repeat opposite side

Cooldown

- ➢ Seated butterfly pose
- ➢ Legs straight; fold
- ➢ Left leg straight, bend right knee; fold to left leg
- ➢ Right leg straight, bend left knee; fold to right leg
- ➢ Lie on belly for sphinx pose
- ➢ Bow pose
- ➢ Lie on back for bridge pose
- ➢ Supine twist, both sides
- ➢ Savasana

Closing Meditation:

To forgive is to reclaim the power that was taken from you when you were hurt, wronged, or abused. Until I forgive someone who has hurt, abused, or wronged me, they take up space in my head and my soul, and in this way they have power over me.

In his book *The Second Mountain: The Quest for a Moral Life*, author David Brooks says that "real forgiveness is rigorous [and] it balances accountability with mercy and compassion." It begins, he says, "with a gesture by the one who has been wronged."[50] In other words, the victim makes the first move because she is the one with the power—the power to forgive. It's now up to the offender to confess, to be remorseful, to be honest, to submit. When the victim and the offender can do these things, it removes the barrier to relationship. It doesn't mean trust is restored or the sin ignored. It does mean, at best, that the victim offers grace and is thus freed from resentment and vengeance. And the offender, made humble, grows as a person because of the experience.

David Brooks's recipe is appealing, and yet for some it is idealistic or unrealistic. It works best when both parties are fully engaged, which we know isn't always the case. So, what can you do as a victim when the offender won't come to the table wholeheartedly? If you are willing, you can undertake your portion of the work to release anger, resentment, and desire for vengeance. You can say a metta meditation once or as many times as it takes to rid yourself of the burden of resentment. In Buddhism, a metta meditation is a simple act of directing benevolence, lovingkindness, and goodwill toward another person. Many people say metta meditations daily.

Invite participants to lie down and make themselves comfortable and warm. The class will move from this meditation into Savasana. Invite them to listen as you say, slowly and reverently:

> Hear and feel these first words for yourself, knowing that you are beloved:
> May I be happy, healthy and whole,
> May I have love, warmth and affection,
> May I be protected from harm and free from fear,
> May I be alive, engaged and joyful
> May I experience inner peace and ease
> May everything I experience today point me toward my highest good.[51]

---

50. David Brooks, *The Second Mountain: The Quest for a Moral Life* (New York: Random House, 2019), 169–60.

51. Adapted from *https://palousemindfulness.com/docs/lovingkindness.pdf*.

Direct these next words to someone—living or dead—who has deeply cared for you. I find that permitting my face to smile while I say these words lights the flame of compassion in my heart:

> May you be happy, healthy and whole,
> May you have love, warmth and affection,
> May you be protected from harm and free from fear,
> May you be alive, engaged and joyful
> May you experience inner peace and ease
> May everything you experience today point you toward your highest good.

The next round of meditation may be directed to others you know—to your community, your neighbors, or even complete strangers if you like. Visualize these people as best as you can. Animals can be included as well—both pets and wild creatures. "May you be happy . . ." [Continue, as above.]

The final round of meditation is directed toward those with whom we've experienced conflict or difficulty. As you feel able, direct these words toward the one who has hurt, abused, or offended you: "May you be happy . . ." [Continue, as above.]

As you rest in Savasana, imagine the love God has for you and for all life. Let it fall on you like a gentle and friendly rain. Let it soak into you. Let it soothe and refresh you. Let it fill your reservoir of peace.

Extras: A beautiful prayer-poem titled "Kuan Yin's Prayer for the Abuser" is readily discoverable online and, printed on good paper, would be a fitting take-home gift. Because this topic inevitably will raise painful, difficult, and even traumatic memories for some, consider including the pastoral office's contact information for those who seek a pastoral conversation, one on one.

Workshop 5: Grief and Loss–How Yoga and Christianity Can Help

Workshop Focus: This workshop, offered in the early months of the pandemic as a strange new spring turned to an equally strange new summer, helped participants put a name to the vague sadness they were experiencing. With some modification of language, the workshop can be adapted to other experiences of loss: loss of health and confidence following a grave medical diagnosis, the loss of a beloved one to death, the loss felt when the last child leaves the nest of home, the loss experienced in divorce. Inviting a trusted grief counselor to participate in the workshop (for example, leading a group conversation after class) can be a healing addition. In advertising this workshop, you may wish to invite participants to bring a favorite lap blanket or pillow. If your church has a prayer shawl ministry, consider inviting them to lend or donate some shawls—or even attend the workshop and knit quietly in pews or chairs set around the perimeter of the gathering as a prayerful and supportive presence.

Music Suggestions:

Peter Gabriel, "With This Love," track 16 on *Passion: Music for the Last Temptation of Christ*, Real World Studios, 1989. (arrival and check in)

Meditative Mind, "Hang Drum and Water Drum," *https://www.meditativemind.org. (opening meditation and flow)*

Dead Can Dance, "Devorzhum," track 8 on *Spiritchaser*, 4AD/Warner Bros. Records, 1996. (closing Savasana)

Pranayama: *Dirga* (three-part breath) pranayama.

Yoga Teachings:

The experience of loss is one of the most important experiences human beings can share. Loss is losing a loved one to death. Loss is also keenly felt when we cannot gather in person to share our sorrow. The inability to gather to celebrate threshold moments like retirements, graduations, weddings, and birth elicits a sense of loss. Even changes in what constitutes "normal life" can lead to a sense of loss.

Loss often brings with it a change of identity. I was a married woman. Now, I am a widow. Relationships, careers, abilities, accomplishments—these all define us. When they are gone, who we are is changed. Because we live in a culture uncomfortable with loss, death, endings, and grief, we may be urged to get back to normal or to move on. Without support, our loss can be amplified by feeling abandoned and alone. It's impossible to move on, for "grief impacts every aspect of our being. It affects us physically, mentally, cognitively, emotionally, spiritually and philosophically, in every aspect of body, mind, and spirit."[52]

Yoga offers resources to help with grief. It reminds us that even though a part of who we are has been lost, we are still whole, and our body, mind, and spirit still dwell in union with one another, with others, with God. Yoga is a gentle, healing practice that allows us to adapt and adjust to a new reality: "Yoga asks us again and again to simply be with what is, with compassion

52. Karla Helbert, *Yoga for Grief and Loss* (London, Signing Dragon, 2016, 16).

toward ourselves and others, being exactly how and where we are in the present moment."[53]

Yoga sutra 1.2 states, "Yogas chitta vritti nirodah," or "When you can control the rising of the mind into ripples, you will experience yoga."[54] This rising of the mind has been called the "monkey mind"—the constant chatter of thinking. While it's impossible to fully turn off thoughts (except perhaps in deep meditation), we can befriend and calm them. Limit news, social media, and contact with negative or demanding people. In quiet, observe your own thoughts without becoming absorbed in them. As a thought arises, ask, "Is it true?" The practice of yoga will continually spiral you back to your true Self.

Yoga reminds us that even in difficult times, we are whole and perfect just as we are. Living through the pandemic, we have experienced a shift in perspective. Things we used to regard as important may no longer have the same value. Conversely, perhaps the smallest things have become more important in life. Yoga instructor and licensed professional therapist Karla Helbert observes, "Knowing that we cannot change reality, we are faced with the task of making our lives conform to a brand new and wholly undesirable normal."[55] We may not be able to fix our current reality, but we can allow ourselves the space to adapt and adjust—to reimagine who we are now with compassion, patience, and kindness for ourselves and others. Yoga asks that of us as it unifies our physical bodies, our minds, and our spirits over and over again through love.

Christian Teachings:

✝ I invite you to close or soften your eyes to receive this meditation: God, the divine web, you order life with roles and places for all that has breath. Hear us, a people disconnected from what binds us together and gives our lives meaning. Witness our pain and confusion. Receive our burdens, and carry the weight of our days. You who make all things new, remake us as you need us to be *now, in this present world*, to do your work. Make us conduits of your grace and will. Light the path before us so we are sure of your presence.

Flutter open your eyes. One kind of loss that many of us are feeling right now is the loss of hopes and dreams, the loss of plans for the future, even the

53. Helbert, *Yoga for Grief and Loss*, 21.

54. *The Yoga Sutras of Patanjali*, 3.

55. Helbert, *Yoga for Grief and Loss*, 20.

loss of our sense of who we are in relation to those dreams. The loss of hopes and dreams is a hard one to bear because dreams have little shape or size until they become reality. Nonetheless, we add to those dreams in our idle hours, and even the simple act of thinking about them makes us happy. Now all of that has been taken away or at least put on indefinite hold. We find ourselves not daring to dream, lest we suffer yet one more disappointment.

I invite you to close or soften your eyes. God, the divine dream-planter, you are the source of all our aspirations and all the good we achieve. Hear us as we lament the loss of our cherished plans and dreams. We bring you our fear of the future and bid you replace it with wonder at the gift of the present moment and with hope for a better day ahead. You whose power moves mountains, help us remember you will never abandon us. Help us see the future as a garden that you and we plant together. Help us to plant our dreams there and to allow you to nurture their growth. Remind us that we draw our most vital identity from you and that we are ever and always your own.

Suggested Asana Flows:

Warm-up

- ➢ Easy seat
- ➢ Seated side bend right, seated side bend left
- ➢ Seated twist right, seated twist left
- ➢ Tabletop
- ➢ Cat-cow
- ➢ Downward-facing dog
- ➢ Lizard, right foot forward
- ➢ Forward fold—halfway lift—forward fold
- ➢ Hands over the head pose
- ➢ Forward fold
- ➢ Plank
- ➢ Downward-facing dog
- ➢ Lizard, left foot forward
- ➢ Forward fold—halfway lift—forward fold
- ➢ Hands over the head pose
- ➢ Forward fold
- ➢ Child's pose

Flow

- ➢ Mountain pose
- ➢ Standing staff, left leg lifted
- ➢ Step back left leg; lower left knee down
- ➢ Low lunge pose; twist to the right
- ➢ Half-splits; straighten the right leg
- ➢ Low lunge pose
- ➢ Lift left knee into high crescent lunge; twist to the right
- ➢ High crescent lunge
- ➢ Pyramid; straighten both legs and fold forward
- ➢ Standing splits; balance on the right leg, lifting the left leg
- ➢ Forward fold
- ➢ Garland pose
- ➢ Hands over head pose
- ➢ Goddess the arms
- ➢ Hands over head pose
- ➢ Twist left, right arm in front, left arm behind
- ➢ Hands over head pose
- ➢ Twist right, left arm in front, right arm behind
- ➢ Hands over head pose
- ➢ Goddess the arms
- ➢ Forward fold
- ➢ Plank
- ➢ Lower down onto belly
- ➢ Baby cobra
- ➢ Child's pose
- ➢ Repeat opposite side

Cooldown

- ➢ Seated butterfly pose
- ➢ Legs straight; fold
- ➢ Left leg straight, bend right knee; fold to left leg
- ➢ Right leg straight, bend left knee; fold to right leg
- ➢ Lie on belly for sphinx pose

- Bow pose
- Lie on back for bridge pose
- Supine twist, both sides
- Savasana

Closing Meditation:

When we are grieving there is something sacred about being held by another human being. No words are necessary. To be held says all that we need to hear, and what we need to hear is that we are not alone in this. Someone is with us. Someone is suffering with us. Someone is in solidarity with us. People of faith—people who believe in a benevolent and loving God—understand that in the absence of human touch, this same sense of being held is available to us always.

As you begin to rest in Savasana, I invite you to call to mind your best memory of being held.

Perhaps you are on your mama's lap, wrapped in a blanket so familiar it is like a part of your own body. Your head rests on your mama's chest, and the very smell of her is comforting. Nothing can harm you here.

Perhaps you are curled before a fire on a cold winter's day, supported by pillows, joined by a beloved dog or cat, snuggled up with a loving spouse or a child. No words are spoken because no words are needed. The flames draw your attention and soften your mind. Your breathing is easy and quiet. Your muscles relax. Your mind slows down to the gentle pace of peace. Nothing can trouble you here.

Perhaps you are floating on the water of your favorite pond in summer. The sun is warm on your face. The wind in the trees whispers to you in friendship. Birds sing, and your mind soars with them, wondering what it is like to be held aloft by the wind. Nothing can call you away from this moment.

Where is that sacred place for you—that place of being held; that place where nothing can harm you, nothing can trouble you, and nothing can call you away? Allow a loving and compassionate God to help you create that space. Relax into it. Be at peace.

Extras: Consider bringing a crockpot, set to "warm" and filled with a supply of damp face cloths sprinkled with a calming (and skin safe) essential oil that can be offered during Savasana. You might include a postworkshop discussion circle with cups of chamomile tea. Or perhaps you offer as take-home gifts small candles tied with raffia and a tag lettered with Jesus's words from Matthew 28:20: "And remember, I am with you always, to the end of the age."

Workshop 6: Fire on the Mountain–Passion and Anger in Yoga and Christianity

Workshop Focus: There's nothing like yoga and Christianity coming together to do a deep dive into a topic that many of us have been taught is verboten. In the church world we talk about leaning in to difficult topics and offering space to talk about things the world seems to want to stow out of sight. If we don't talk about anger and passion—and claim them as a part of being human, part of being made in the divine image—then we end up confused by (and distrustful of) a God who in scripture displays both.

In your advertising for this workshop, be clear that the intent is to draw these topics into the light and look more closely at them. Be aware that someone with anger management issues usually leaves in their wake people traumatized by their anger. Your workshop may draw some of those traumatized victims who are seeking to make sense of things. It could also possibly attract people who themselves struggle to contain their anger. Be prepared. Be sensitive. Be supportive. The goal of this workshop is to consider this question: Can anger and passion serve a healthy purpose? Be aware that some people may struggle to consider that question.

Music Suggestions:

Peter Gabriel, "With This Love," track 16 on *Passion: Music for the Last Temptation of Christ*, Real World Studios, 1989. (arrival and check in)

Kenneth Soares, "Activate Qi Flow with Om Mantra & Drums," PowerThoughts Meditation Club, 2015. (opening meditation and flow) *https://insighttimer.com/kennethsoares/guided-meditations/activate-qi-flow-with-om-mantra-and-drums*

Paul Winter, "Nevaga," track 7 on *Solstice Live!*, Living Music, 1993. (closing Savasana)

Pranayama: *Bastrika* breath.

Yoga Teachings:

Patanjali's yoga sutra 1.2 states that yoga is the cessation of the modifications, or fluctuations of the mind. The study and practice of yoga and its eight limbs invites the exploration of the emotional fluctuations and modifications of the mind. This is the "mind chatter" that pulls us away from the present moment and traps us in an endless cycle of thinking. We are distracted, unable to focus on what is before us. We ruminate. Yoga provides the tools to quiet and calm the mind. It can assist us in avoiding impulsive, anger-driven behavior and poor decision-making that cause harm to others or ourselves. It can also assist us in dealing with negative emotions in the moment instead of suppressing them, only to have them surprise us later.

According to yogic philosophy, anger arises because of the predominance of the powerful rajasic energy. Rajasic energy is important because it helps us take action and accomplish things. But too much rajasic energy can lead to aggressive behavior and negative and destructive manifestations of anger. According to yoga theory,

> While anger can be beneficial if expressed and addressed appropriately, uncontrolled anger negatively affects not only the mind, but also the physical body and relationships. Anger triggers the fight-or-flight response, which floods the body with stress hormones, and the long-term physical effects of uncontrolled anger include anxiety, depression, high blood pressure, headache, heart attack, and decreased immune response.
>
> Uncontrolled anger directly competes with the yogic principle of Ahimsa, or nonviolence toward all living things, and can lead to trouble at work, arguments, physical fights, and emotionally pushing people away.[56]

In this workshop we use pranayama, asana, svadhyaya, and tapas to better understand the source of our anger and to learn to channel its energy in nondestructive ways. Using these yogic tools will, over time, help quiet the mind and promote greater self-awareness and self-control.

The Sanskrit word *akrodha* means "without or absence of anger." Akrodha is considered a virtue and high ethical value. When someone is insulted or provoked, akrodha means being calm and nonreactive, keeping an even temper despite the circumstances. When we attain akrodha, we can face obstacles and challenges without anger and greet them instead with a productive, positive, and constructive state of mind: "Dharma, our purpose in life, relies on akrodha, because it creates an environment of serenity, a rational principle of life, and because it is a moral virtue inspired by love."[57] One of the Upanishads (ancient texts of India) teaches, "All cruel words should be endured. None should be treated with disrespect. No anger should be directed in turn towards one who is angry. Only soft words should be spoken, even when violently pulled by another."[58]

---

56. Ling Beisecker, "5 Yogic Ways to Manage and Deal with Anger," Do You, accessed October 21, 2021, *https://www.doyouyoga.com/5-yogic-ways-to-manage-and-deal-with-anger-52744/*.

57. Wikipedia, s.v. "Akrodha," last modified July 5, 2021, *https://en.wikipedia.org/wiki/Akrodha*.

58. K. Narayanasvami Aiyar, *Narada Parivrajaka Upanishad of Atharva Veda*, 1914, chapter 3, *https://www.wisdomlib.org/hinduism/book/narada-parivrajaka-upanishad-of-atharvaveda/d/doc217045.html*.

Another ancient text, the Hindu epic *Mahabharata*, emphasizes the virtue of akrodha and the niyama of ahimsa, which is nonviolence toward the Self and others. The epic states, "If wronged, you should not wrong in return. One's anger, if not subdued, burns one's own self; if subdued, it procures the virtues of the doers of good acts. You should never give pain to others by cruel words. Never defeat your enemies by despicable means. Never utter sinful and burning words as may give pain to others."[59]

The *Mahabharata* also teaches:

> Anger is in this world, the root of the destruction of mankind. The angry person commits a sin; the angry person murders their preceptor; the angry person insults with harsh words. The angry person cannot distinguish what should be and should not be said by them; there is nothing which cannot be said or done by an angry person. From anger, a person may kill one who should not be killed and adore one that should be slain; an angry person may even despatch their own self to the abode of Yama. Beholding these evils, anger must be conquered."[60]

Here is a story about Kali, the Hindu goddess of war, anger, and destruction.

Once upon a time, the god Shiva, the lord of destruction, was so busy meditating that he was not doing his godly duties on earth. The other gods petitioned the great goddess Kali to manifest as Sati, a beautiful woman who would become Shiva's wife and draw him back into engagement with the world. She agreed to do so and took on a minor god, Daksha, as her father, so long as no one ever forgot who she really was. Daksha gained enough power as a religious leader that he started to think himself more powerful than his daughter, Sati, and her husband, Shiva, whom he disliked. He held a great fire ceremony and invited everyone in the godly universe but Shiva and Sati. This was a grave mistake. Daksha was so preoccupied with the trappings of his ceremony he forgot that his very daughter was the manifestation of Shakti Kali, the reason for all religion. He broke his promise to her, that who she really was would never be forgotten.

When Sati found out what Daksha had done, she was infuriated. She told Shiva she was going to go confront her father, and Shiva, who had little time for religious showmanship, told her to calm down. At that, Sati did what most

59. Vyasa Mahabarata, *Adi Parva*, chapter 87, verses 7–8, *https://en.wikipedia.org/wiki/Akrodha*.

60. Vyasa Mahabarata, *Vana Parva*, chapter 29, verses 3–7, *https://en.wikipedia.org/wiki/Akrodha*.

angry people do when they are told to calm down: she got angrier. Shiva lost his patience. "I forbid it!" he said. At that, Sati turned black. Her fangs came out, and her mouth dripped with blood. Her long black hair grew wild and unkempt, a necklace of severed male heads appeared around her neck, and a huge sharp sword appeared in her hand. "You forbid it?" she asked quietly. Terrified, Shiva tried to run away, but everywhere he turned a new fierce goddess appeared, blocking his way. "Where is my beautiful Sati?" he cried. "Right in front of you," said this dark goddess, whose name was Kali. "This is my true face. I only appear beautiful and sweet as a favor to you. If you ever try to control me again, I will fight you in this form." Shiva recognized the power of his wife and got the hell out of her way.

Kali is one of the most popular goddesses in India. She is the great destroyer, even more powerful than her husband, Shiva, and in her destruction, she allows new things to be born. In this way, she is both a killer and a mother. She's sometimes understood as the shadow side of life (like anger or death) that we don't want to look in the face. But as she tells Shiva, her fierce, bloody face is her true self. Death is a reality of life. Anger and rage can reveal whatever truth has been bubbling beneath the surface.

We reveal prettier faces to the world most of the time because we catch more flies with honey. Love and forgiveness are powerful too. But we must not forget the Kali that lives inside each of us. Rage can give us the strength to see past fear and take action. Every now and then we need to rise up, bare our true fangs, and resist.[61]

Pranayama allows us to access our breath. Svadhyaya encourages us to engage in the self-study of anger—learning where it comes from and diving deeper into the reasons for our feelings and reactions. A third yogic resource is tapas. Tapas is a fire within us that translates as "austerity" or "discipline," and it means to burn or to purify. When we tap into our tapas, we light our inner fire. This enables us to cultivate a sense of self-discipline, passion, and courage to burn away "impurities" of physical, mental, and emotional mind chatter—including anger. Tapas is a fierceness that gets our heart pumping and heightens our desire for personal growth. It has the power to change us and pave the way to our intrinsic greatness, our true Self. Tapas is used in all aspects of yoga practice, both on and off our mats.

61. Derived from Julie Peters, "Kali, Goddess of Rage and Resistance," Spirituality and Health, accessed October 21, 2021, *https://spiritualityhealth.com/blogs/downward-blog-a-life-in-yoga/2017/06/08/julie-peters-kali-goddess-rage-and-resistance#*.

Tapas is a niyama, a moral and ethical observance. By practicing niyamas, or observances, we cultivate a deeper understanding of how to live our yoga practice off the mat and begin to make real changes to our lives.

Christian Teachings:

✝ Anger is "a response to a perceived threat to oneself or to another. It is a response to frustration."[62] Frustration is what happens when you do something and expect a given reward or outcome but it doesn't happen. Repeated frustration can lead to anger.

Poet David Whyte says that if you strip away violence from anger, you're left with "the purest form of care. The internal living flame of anger always illuminates what we belong to, what we wish to protect and what we are willing to hazard ourselves for." He says that "what we name as anger is actually only the incoherent physical incapacity to sustain this deep form of care in our daily life; the unwillingness to be large enough and generous enough to hold what we love helplessly in our bodies or our mind with the clarity and breadth of our whole being."[63] Anger has also been called a "disordered love"—in other words, a good emotion gone bad.[64]

Anger presents an opportunity for spiritual growth. It's been said that "the most important type of spiritual growth doesn't happen when you're meditating or on a yoga mat. It happens in the midst of conflict—when you're frustrated, angry, or scared and you're doing the same old thing, and then you suddenly realize you have a choice to do it differently."[65]

✝ We're culturally conditioned to be embarrassed for getting angry, because it usually represents a loss of control. For many years social scientists have regarded anger as "a vestige from our savage past that serve[s] no useful purpose in contemporary life." They "thought anger was [an embarrassing emotion] that mature people and societies ought to suppress." That attitude began to shift in the 1970s, when researchers found that anger is actually "one of the

---

62. *https://www.ncbi.nlm.nih.gov/pmc/articles/PMC3260787/* and L. Berkowitz, *Aggression: Its Causes, Consequences, and Control* (Philadelphia: Temple University Press, 1993).

63. David Whyte, *Consolations: The Solace, Nourishment and Underlying Meaning of Everyday Words* (Langley, WA: Many Rivers Press, 2015), 13–15.

64. William S. Stafford, *Disordered Loves: Healing the Seven Deadly Sins* (Boston: Cowley Publications, 1994).

65. Chocolako, "Spiritual Growth Does Not Happen When We Are Meditating," *Elephant Journal*, September 8, 2019, *https://www.elephantjournal.com/2019/09/spiritual-growth-does-not-happen-when-we-are-meditating-chocolako/*.

densest forms of communication. It conveys more information, more quickly, than almost any other type of emotion. And it does an excellent job of forcing us to listen to and confront problems we might otherwise avoid."[66]

Anger has some purpose: it can motivate us to undertake difficult tasks. We're often more creative when we're angry, because our outrage helps us see solutions we've overlooked. When researchers studied "the brains of people who [were] expressing anger, they [looked] very similar to people who [were] experiencing happiness."[67]

Anger used well can effect positive social change: Dr. Martin Luther King Jr. taught that being angry is not enough. You can't just release your emotion by hurling insults and then retreat into smug, passive satisfaction. "The supreme task," said King, "is to organize and unite people so that their anger becomes a transforming force."[68] In the Bible, God's anger arises most often because God sees injustice. Anger used well can inspire people to action to right a wrong, to work for justice and peace and for the dignity of all life. Theologian William Stafford said that "the love of social justice is . . . anger transposed to a higher level." It's a motivation to guard "everyone's integrity and essential needs [and] not just one's own."[69]

✝ Anger and the desire for revenge are not the same thing: "Ordinary anger can deepen, under the right circumstances, into moral indignation—a more combustible form of the emotion, though one that can still be a powerful force for good. If moral indignation persists, however—and if the indignant lose faith that their anger is being heard—it can produce a third type of anger: a desire for revenge against our enemies that privileges inflicting punishment over reaching accord."[70] Though anger and the desire for revenge can feel intertwined, they are two distinct emotions. Simply becoming angry doesn't prompt a revenge impulse. Can you think of anger as a cleansing fire and the desire for revenge as a sludge that clogs the workings of the soul?

✝ The Bible advises we should be slow to anger: "Whoever is slow to anger has great understanding, but one who has a hasty temper exalts folly" (Prov.

66. Charles Duhigg, "The Real Roots of American Rage," *The Atlantic*, January/February 2019, *https://www.theatlantic.com/magazine/archive/2019/01/charles-duhigg-american-anger/576424/*.

67. Duhigg, "The Real Roots of American Rage."

68. Duhigg, "The Real Roots of American Rage."

69. Stafford, *Disordered Loves*, 77.

70. Duhigg, "The Real Roots of American Rage."

14:29). "Know this, my beloved brothers: let every person be quick to hear, slow to speak, slow to anger" (James 1:19 ESV). We're to follow the example of God, who is "merciful and gracious, slow to anger and abounding in steadfast love" (Ps. 103:8). The Bible doesn't say, "God *never* gets angry." It says instead two things: first, God is *slow* to get angry; and second, that God's mercy, graciousness, and abundant, enduring love better describe God than does anger.

Listening—and really listening well—seems to be tied to our ability to be slow to anger. There is great value in listening and investigating before rushing to judgment. Acting on angry impulse leads to nothing good. It leaves us vulnerable and makes fools of us. I appreciate how Proverbs 25:28 ESV puts it: "A man without self-control is like a city broken into and left without walls."

In the New Testament, Paul offers some more advice in Ephesians 4:26: "Be angry but do not sin; do not let the sun go down on your anger." What's interesting is that Paul isn't telling his listeners not to be angry. He's instead cautioning them not to let their anger cause them to do something foolish and hurtful. He is counseling them not to make room in themselves for anger to become a long-term guest: "Do not let the sun go down on your anger." Why would that be? Because to harbor anger is corrosive to the soul. An unsourced saying attributed to the first-century Roman Stoic philosopher Lucius Annaeus Seneca (Seneca the Younger) observes, "Anger is an acid that can do more harm to the vessel in which it is stored than to anything on which it is poured."

✝ Nahum 1:2–6 ESV is a rich description of God's anger:

> The LORD is a jealous and avenging God;
> the LORD is avenging and wrathful;
> the LORD takes vengeance on his adversaries
> and keeps wrath for his enemies.
> The LORD is slow to anger and great in power,
> and the LORD will by no means clear the guilty.
> His way is in whirlwind and storm,
> and the clouds are the dust of his feet.
> He rebukes the sea and makes it dry;
> he dries up all the rivers;
> Bashan and Carmel wither;
> the bloom of Lebanon withers.
> The mountains quake before him;
> the hills melt;

the earth heaves before him,
  the world and all who dwell in it.
Who can stand before his indignation?
  Who can endure the heat of his anger?
His wrath is poured out like fire,
  and the rocks are broken into pieces by him.

Ashamed Christians have tried to distance themselves from these depictions of God's wrath and have tried to explain them away. But as creatures made in the divine image, it's important for us to acknowledge that we have anger and God does too.

Why is God angry in scripture? Often it is because God is jealous or exasperated: the people are worshiping idols instead of God, or they are stubborn and stiff-necked and refuse to listen to God, or they are selfish and hypocritical instead of being compassionate and generous. Theologian William Stafford wrote, "Right anger is commitment to integrity and the social fabric, not the reverse. It acts to defend life and justice. In this sense it is possible to be angry in love."[71] Given this, I invite you to consider the possibility in scripture that God is angry because God is committed to integrity and the social fabric, because God wishes to defend life and justice. In short, God is sometimes angry because God loves.

✝ In scripture, fire is often a metaphor for passion. (For a parallel concept in yoga, see definitions and discussions of tapas.) In scripture, fire is also a vehicle through which God interacts with humans. The biblical writers used fire to describe God's body parts (his mouth, voice, and legs) to anthropomorphize him—to give God human qualities so we humans can better grasp the concept of God. And yet, no human emits fire, so describing God as fiery sets God apart as not human. God is humanlike but not human. Fire is dangerous and lethal if you engage with it carelessly. Fire is also purifying and life-sustaining if you engage with it properly. Scripture seems to employ fire to say these same things about God.[72]

Several places in the New Testament link fire and passion. In Luke 12:49–56, Jesus declares that he came to bring fire to the earth. He goes on to speak about how he didn't come to bring peace to the earth but rather division. This is a difficult saying, and one scholar suggests that the fire Jesus is talking about is

---

71. Stafford, *Disordered Loves*, 77.

72. Dr. Deenah Grant, "God's Flaming Fiery Anger," The Torah, accessed October 21, 2021, https://*www.thetorah.com/article/gods-flaming-fiery-anger*.

passion—ardor, or a burning love for God.[73] Jesus wishes it was already kindled; if nothing else it would make his job much easier. Anyone who's built a fire knows it's easier to start one with a burning ember and kindling than it is cold, dead logs. Perhaps one interpretation is that the people's hearts are those cold, dead logs. Jesus will have to work like crazy to get them stirred up with passion for God.

In Matthew 13:13, Jesus tells his disciples they are the salt of the earth but that if salt loses its taste, it's good for nothing. The implication is that if the disciples lose their passion, their internal fire, they are useless. In the book of Revelation, the Lord sends a message to one of the churches and says, "'I know your works; you are neither cold nor hot. I wish that you were either cold or hot! So, because you are lukewarm, and neither hot nor cold, I am about to spit you out of my mouth" (3:15–16). In other words, without passion and internal fire, the church is useless.

Finally, a Christian parallel to the yogic concept of tapas can be found in the writings of the twelfth-century Christian mystic Hildegard of Bingen. She recorded a vision in which God said to her, "I, the highest and fiery power, have kindled every spark of life. . . . I, the fiery life of divine essence, am aflame beyond the beauty of the meadows, I gleam in the waters, and I burn in the sun, moon, and stars. . . . I remain hidden in every kind of reality as a fiery power. Everything burns because of me in the way our breath constantly moves us, like the wind-tossed flame in a fire."[74]

Suggested Asana Flows:

Warm-up

- ➢ Mountain pose
- ➢ Side bend left, side bend right
- ➢ Chair pose
- ➢ Standing staff, left leg lifted
- ➢ Step left leg back into warrior I
- ➢ Plank
- ➢ Lower down onto belly
- ➢ Baby cobra

---

73. Lauren F. Winner, *Wearing God: Clothing, Laughter, Fire, and Other Overlooked Ways of Meeting God* (New York: HarperOne, 2015), 204–5.

74. Winner, *Wearing God*, 205.

- Downward-facing dog
- Forward fold—halfway lift—forward fold
- Hands over head pose
- Side bend left, side bend right
- Chair pose
- Standing staff, right leg lifted
- Step right leg back into warrior I
- Plank
- Lower down onto belly
- Baby cobra
- Child's pose

Flow

- Tabletop
- Cat-cow
- Bird dog, left leg back and right arm forward
- Gate pose, left leg, left side
- Side plank, right hand and knee down, left leg up
- Tabletop
- Cat-cow
- Bird dog, right leg back and left arm forward
- Gate pose, right leg, right side
- Side plank, left hand and knee down, right leg up
- Tabletop
- Downward-facing dog
- Warrior 1, right foot forward
- Humble warrior
- Bound warrior III
- Warrior I
- Extended side angle
- Reverse triangle
- Half moon balance on right leg, right arm down
- Release to forward fold
- Plank

- Lower down onto belly
- Baby cobra
- Downward-facing dog
- Repeat opposite side

Cooldown

- Tabletop
- Sleeping pigeon, right leg forward
- Half frog, right knee bent as release from pigeon
- Climbing tree frog, left arm toward top of mat; twist right to look to ceiling
- Tabletop
- Sleeping pigeon, left leg forward
- Half frog, left knee bent as release from pigeon
- Climbing tree frog, right arm toward top of mat; twist left to look to ceiling
- Locust
- Roll over to back
- Stretch through fingertips and toes
- Boat pose
- Supine twist, both sides
- Savasana

Closing Meditation (Options):

✤ Offer this prayer from the fourteenth-century Christian mystic Catherine of Siena: "You, God, are a fire that always burns without consuming. You are a fire consuming in its heat every compartment of the soul's self-absorbed love. You are a fire lifting all chill and giving all light. In Your light You show me Your truth. You're the Light that outshines every Light."[75]

God is a fire that consumes in its heat every compartment of the soul's self-absorbed love. When that self-absorbed love has been consumed, what remains is outward-facing love: love for the divine, love for others, and, finally, compassion and kind regard for the Self.

75. Christine Valters Paintner, *Water, Wind, Earth, and Fire: The Christian Practice of Praying with the Elements* (Notre Dame, IN: Sorin Books, 2010), 55.

✝ Offer this from the twentieth-century Christian mystic Pierre Teilhard de Chardin: "The day will come when after we have mastered the winds, the waves, the tides, and gravity, we shall harness for God the energies of love. Then for the second time in the history of the world, [humankind] will have discovered fire."[76]

Fire, passion, tapas, love. These all carry the energy of the divine. May they carry you into the days ahead.

Offer this story while participants are in Savasana: A Hindu saint visited the river Ganges to take a bath and found a group of family members on the banks, shouting in anger at each other. He turned to his disciples, smiled, and asked, "Why do people shout in anger at each other?" The disciples thought for a while, and one of them said, "Because we lose our calm, we shout."

"But why should you shout when the other person is just next to you? You can as well tell him what you have to say in a soft manner," asked the Hindu saint. The disciples offered some other answers, but none satisfied the saint.

Finally, the saint explained, "When two people are angry at each other, their hearts distance a lot. To cover that distance, they must shout to be able to hear each other. The angrier they are, the stronger they will have to shout to hear each other to cover that great distance. What happens when two people fall in love? They don't shout at each other, but talk softly, because their hearts are very close. The distance between them is either nonexistent or very small."

The saint continued, "When they love each other even more, what happens? They do not speak, only whisper, and they get even closer to each other in their love. Finally, they even need not whisper; they need only look at each other. That is how close two people are when they love each other."

He looked at his disciples and said, "So when you argue do not let your hearts get distant, do not say words that distance each other more, or else there will come a day when the distance is so great that you will not find the path to return."[77]

Bring students slowly out of Savasana and into a seated position with hands at heart center in anjali mudra (prayer position).

Extras: Send participants home with a taper candle, with one of the closing meditation prayers tied to it as a tag. When setting up for this workshop, if it can be safely done, consider adding burning candles to the worship space.

76. Paintner, *Water, Wind, Earth, and Fire*, 62.

77. "Why We Shout When in Anger—A Hindu Spiritual Story," Spiritual Growth Events, accessed October 21, 2021, *http://www.spiritual-short-stories.com/spiritual-short-story-505-why-we-shout-when-in-anger/*.

Workshop 7: Standing on Holy Ground–Yoga and Christianity Converse about the Divine in Creation

Workshop Focus: If you were to ask people where God lives, the most likely answer you'd receive is "in heaven." When last surveyed, over 70 percent of Americans believe heaven is a place where people who lived good lives are eternally rewarded.[78] If you pressed and asked where heaven is located, most people would answer that heaven is in the sky or the clouds, or beyond. They wouldn't be wrong, exactly, because the Bible describes heaven in this way. In fact, both the Hebrew and Greek words for "heaven" can also be translated as "sky."[79] Is beyond the clouds the *only* place God lives? This workshop suggests it is merely one among countless places where God can be found.

At St. John's, we offered this workshop during the week of Earth Day in April. It's an ideal workshop to offer outdoors at the church or even in a meadow or woods with ample flat ground. If held indoors in the worship space, open the windows.

Once you start searching the Bible with an eye toward finding God in creation, there's enough material for an entire series: God in the wind, God in the water, God in the soil and growing things, God in fire. Contemporary theologians in the tradition of Celtic spirituality, like John Philip Newell, or in creation theology, like Matthew Fox, provide abundant material for such a series. Also look to medieval mystics, like Hildegard of Bingen, and twentieth-century theologian-scientists, like Pierre Teilhard de Chardin and John Polkinghorne. And do not overlook the writings of Ilia Delio, contemporary scientist-theologian and founder of the Center for Christogenesis.[80] One could teach every week for a year with reflections on the divine in creation without running out of material.

Music Suggestions:

Peter Gabriel, "With This Love," track 16 on *Passion: Music for the Last Temptation of Christ*, Real World Studios, 1989. (arrival and check in)

Sequentia, *Canticles of Ecstasy*, Deutsche Harmonia Mundi, 1993. (opening meditation and flow)

---

78. Caryle Murphy, "Most Americans Believe in Heaven . . . and Hell," Pew Research Center, November 10, 2015, *https://www.pewresearch.org/fact-tank/2015/11/10/most-americans-believe-in-heaven-and-hell/*.

79. Robyn J. Whitaker, "What and Where Is Heaven? The Answers Are at the Heart of the Easter Story," The Conversation, April 18, 2019, *https://theconversation.com/what-and-where-is-heaven-the-answers-are-at-the-heart-of-the-easter-story-115451*.

80. "About the Center for Christogenesis," Center for Christogenesis, accessed October 21, 2021, *https://christogenesis.org/about/*.

Simon Lockyer, "Natural World," track 2 on *Antenatal Relaxation*, Angelworks, 2007. (closing Savasana)

Also search online for sound files from the natural world: waves breaking on a beach, birdsong, a running brook, and so on.

Pranayama: *Dirga* (three-part) breath.

Yoga Teachings:

The string theory of physics (for more, see the following Christian teachings) asserts the world is comprised of vibrating, quivering strings. In your imagination, picture these strings connecting everything on earth, alive and material. These strings have a distinct connection with the yoga sutras. Sutras are considered "strings" or "threads," weaving together the teachings of yogic philosophy. Yoga means to "yoke and unionize" or "bring together, attach" the body, mind, and spirit. It is believed that the body, mind, and spirit are all made up of the elements of nature; we are all created in the same elements of the divine. These elements are believed to represent every possible form of matter: earth, water, fire, air, and space (ether).[81]

Yoga began thousands of years ago as an oral tradition, passed down through many lineages in the language of Sanskrit. Sanskrit is considered the vibrational language of the universe because it has a deep relationship with the divine nature of creation. It is said to mimic the sounds of nature and be directly connected to God. If you have ever participated in chanting, or kirtan, you may have experienced this vibrational flow of the language through the use of your own voice or by feeling in your body the sounds of the voices of others. Chanting Om—especially what's called "the rolling Om"—is a beautiful, physical experience of sound. Om is said to be the sound of the start of the universe. As such, it has a healing frequency.

In yoga, many of the asanas, mudras, mantras, and breathwork are named after things in the natural world. Consider asana names like lizard, fish, tree, mountain, eagle, and heron. Yoga honors the cycles of nature through sun and moon salutations. In pranayama, some examples of nature names are moon breath, sun breath, balancing the sun and moon breath, bee's breath, and fire breath. Ayurveda, which is the sister to yoga, is an ancient holistic whole-body healing system. It recognizes the body to have two sides ruled by the sun (right, masculine) and by the moon (left, feminine). Ayurveda aims to balance the sun and the moon through nature and yoga.

81. Nicolai Bachman, *The Language of Yoga: Complete A-to-Y Guide to Asana Names, Sanskrit Terms, and Chants* (Louisville, CO: Sounds True, 2005).

Yoga seeks to honor and respect the divine in the natural world and in ourselves. It unites our body, mind, and spirit through breath, meditation, and asana, using these bodily temples we were given by God. A sacred mantra, considered the mother of all mantras, gives reverence to the divine in creation. It is dedicated to Savitri (a form of Saraswati), the goddess of the five elements.[82] It is called the Gayatri Mantra. Different translations of it may be found online. Here is one:

Tuning to the elements
Sun, Moon, planets
To the coming and going and balance of life
May you be inspired and guided through the journey of life.

We meditate on the unity of Divine Spirit, which permeates everything,
On Earth, the atmosphere, and the heavens.
May this Supreme Consciousness guide and protect us, and illuminate
Our hearts and our minds.

Gayatri Mantra
Om bhur bhuvah svaha
Tat savitur varenyam
Bhargo devasya dhimahi
Dhiyo yonah prachodayat[83]

Christian Teachings:

✝ What does it mean for the ground to be called *holy*? The term *holy ground* comes from the third chapter of the book of Exodus. In that story, the Israelites are enslaved in Egypt. Moses is out "beyond the wilderness" tending sheep when God speaks to him and tells him to lead the Israelites out of Egypt, out of slavery. The way God manifests is by setting a bush on fire. God—the burning bush—blazes away, waiting for Moses to notice. When Moses does, God speaks and calls to him by name: "Moses, Moses!" "Here I am," says Moses, and God replies, "Stop right there. Take off your sandals, for the place on which you are standing is holy ground."

Wherever we notice the beauty and majesty of the divine, wherever we are standing or sitting at that moment, it is holy ground. All ground is holy if we understand that God is both transcendent *and* immanent. God is transcendent,

82. Wikipedia, s.v. "Gayatri Mantra," last modified October 18, 2021, *https://en.wikipedia.org/wiki/Gayatri_Mantra*.

83. Roger Gabriel, "The Gayatri Mantra for Enlightenment," April 24, 2019, *https://chopra.com/articles/the-gayatri-mantra-for-enlightenment*.

unknowable, far away, vast. God is also immanent, relational, everywhere, and in all things. God is even in those places where you wouldn't expect to find God. The text from Exodus describes Moses as being "beyond the wilderness." You can also translate that as "beyond the uninhabited wasteland"—a very arid, lifeless place, and yet even so, God is there.

✝ Progressive, mystical Christianity acknowledges and celebrates the presence, the essence, the spark of the divine in all matter. It can be easy enough to grasp that concept when you speak of animate matter—creatures that have breath; creatures that transform things like air, sunlight, nutrients into life-sustaining fuel; creatures like fish and eagles and giraffes and even plants.

It's a bit harder to imagine that the divine is present in *inanimate* matter like rocks or clay or dust, but a quantum physicist would suggest that beneath the molecular level of electrons, quarks, and neutrinos, all matter is comprised of quivering strings. Everything—from the yoga mat you are sitting on to the lungs with which you are breathing—is comprised of these strings. It is their vibrational pattern and frequency that determines what or how they manifest. In other words, according to the theory, the superstrings in the yoga mat vibrate at a different frequency and pattern than do the ones in your lungs. The frequency and pattern of the vibration of the superstrings determines the nature of the matter they manifest.[84] What if, just *what if,* those superstrings are how God operates in the world? What a great hiding place for God, being at the ultramicroscopic level of matter!

Norman MacLeod, a nineteenth-century Presbyterian minister from Scotland, taught about the nearness of God in all things: "In the midst of the change and movement and flow of life, in the rising of the morning sun, in the work and relationships of daily life, in the great struggles of society and nation, in alertness to the interior life of the soul, in times of rest and sleep and even dreaming."[85] His prayer, based on the hymn text of *St. Patrick's Breastplate*, prefigures string theory: "Invisible we see you, Christ beneath us. With earthly eyes we see beneath us stones and dust and dross. . . . But with the eyes of faith, we know you uphold. In you all things consist and hold together. The very atom is light energy, the grass is vibrant, the rocks pulsate. All is in flux; turn but a stone and an angel moves."[86]

---

84. Paramahansa Yogananda, *The Yoga of Jesus: Understanding the Hidden Teachings of the Gospels* (Los Angeles: Self-Realization Fellowship, 2007), 26.

85. J. Philip Newell, *Listening for the Heartbeat of God: A Celtic Spirituality* (Mahwah, NJ: Paulist Press, 1997), 76.

86. Newell, *Listening for the Heartbeat of God*, 85.

Even though God is often described as omnipresent (present everywhere), many of us tend to think of God as located above us, spatially speaking. But science-informed theology suggests God is *also* beneath, and among, and within us. It's a different way of understanding the presence of the divine in all creation. There is nothing that does not contain within it something of God. What does this understanding of God mean for how you will be in relationship with the earth? Jesus was fond of saying, "Whatever you do to the vulnerable (the poor, the hungry, the sick, the imprisoned, the voiceless) you do also to me." Consider that whatever you and I do to the vulnerable earth, we do also to God.

✢ Yoga teachers speak endlessly about being grounded, about grounding one's feet or hands or sitz bones into the mat. What yogis call *grounding* some scientists call *earthing*. The surface of the earth offers up a limitless supply of free or mobile electrons. In the course of living, our bodies amass something called *free radicals*. You've likely heard of these. Essentially, they are electrons without a partner—electrons like to be in pairs—and these free radical electrons roam the body seeking a friend. They can do a lot of cell damage as they travel, so it's no surprise that free radicals have been implicated in inflammation, aging, and disease.[87]

When we connect our bodies, our bare skin, to the surface of the earth—the ground—we are able to absorb the earth's mobile electrons. Those electrons carry a *negative* charge. In our bodies, some—not all, but some—of the free radicals carry a *positive* charge. So, an electron from the earth with its negative charge enters the body, meets up with a free radical electron with a positive charge, and—eureka—the free radical is neutralized. The two meet, and it's a love story with a healthy outcome.

Most of us are so far removed from beneficial contact with the earth that we abound in free radicals. We insulate our bodies from contact with the earth with layer upon layer of rubber, plastic, composite material, sealed concrete, and asphalt.

Many of us live bearing the burden of chronic pain, poor sleep, inflammation, chronic stress or anxiety, and disease. It's fascinating and theologically significant that one way toward better health is to simply place our bare feet on the earth, or our hands in the soil of a garden as often as we can.[88] If the divine

---

87. Jessie Szalay, "What Are Free Radicals?" Live Science, May 27, 2016, *https://www.livescience.com/54901-free-radicals.html.*

88. Gaétan Chevalier et al., "Earthing: Health Implications of Reconnecting the Human Body to the Earth's Surface Electrons," *Journal of Environmental Public Health* 2012 (2012): *https://www.ncbi.nlm.nih.gov/pmc/articles/PMC3265077/.*

is in all things, then God is in the earth—in the surface of the earth—and the healing energy of God is readily available to us. Indeed, God created us to receive healing from the earth. In Hebrew, the word for Adam, the first human, is *Adamah*, or "earth creature." From the very beginning we were created to be connected or grounded to the earth.

Suggested Asana Flows:

Warm-up

- ➢ Mountain pose
- ➢ Hands over head pose
- ➢ Anjali mudra at heart center
- ➢ Hands over head pose
- ➢ Forward fold—halfway lift—forward fold
- ➢ Plank
- ➢ Baby cobra
- ➢ Downward-facing dog
- ➢ Tabletop
- ➢ Cat-cow

Flow

- ➢ Downward-facing dog
- ➢ High crescent lunge, right leg forward
- ➢ High crescent lunge with arms lifted, then cactus arms, arms lifted, then airplane arms; bend at waist, arms lifted
- ➢ Warrior II
- ➢ Reverse warrior
- ➢ Pyramid
- ➢ Warrior III, balance on right
- ➢ Forward fold—halfway lift—forward fold
- ➢ Plank
- ➢ Baby cobra
- ➢ Downward-facing dog
- ➢ Repeat opposite side

Cooldown

- ➢ Tabletop
- ➢ Bird dog, right arm forward and left leg back; switch sides
- ➢ Cat-cow
- ➢ Lie on back and squeeze legs into belly
- ➢ Supine twist both sides
- ➢ Savasana

Closing Meditation:

Invite participants to lie down in Savasana. In this guided meditation we begin by relaxing the body, one part at a time, beginning with the toes, then the feet, ankles, calves, knees, thighs, hips, abdomen, ribs, fingers, wrists, arms, shoulders, neck, eyes, lips—in whatever order your yoga teacher typically guides participants.

Call to mind a favorite place on this earth, a place where perhaps you ran barefoot as a child. It could be a meadow, a sandy beach, smooth rocks on the shore of a lake, the cool dark woods, a favorite park, backyard, or garden.

Take a moment and let a picture of that place form in your mind. Smell the air. Notice what the wind is doing. Is it still, or is there a breeze? Feel the sun or the rain on your skin. Without moving your toes, feel them sink into the surface of the earth. Feel the earth meet you and rise up into you. Feel the connection between you and the earth. Can you begin to imagine an exchange of energy taking place?

Begin to feel that earth energy from your favorite place as a warm, luminous, liquid light. Feel it flow into you through the soles of your feet. Let it fill the feet with healing energy. Allow it to rise to the ankles, wrapping them in light. Feel it filling the calves of your legs, rising above the knees, feet, ankles, knees, and legs. This liquid light gently wraps your hips like a shimmering golden cloth. Feel it slowly rise to fill your torso, wave upon wave, filling legs, hips, and torso. As it rises, feel it warm your chest and rest gently upon your shoulders. Torso, chest, and shoulders. The light spirals and flows down your arms to your wrists. Shoulders, arms, and wrists. Feel it pool in your hands, your fingers, your finger-tips. Feel it travel softly like liquid up your back, to your neck, feel it bathe your head in warm, luminous, liquid light. The light of the healing energy of the earth. Divine presence. Healing light. Rest now in that light.

Extras: Consider sending participants home with a tangible reminder of the divine in creation: a smooth stone, shell, feather, small potted plant, small jar or bottle of stream or spring water that has been blessed. Add a verse from scripture, one of these teachings, or a poem that will remind participants to take what they learned home with them.

Workshop 8: Pay Attention—What Yoga and Christianity Have to Say about Living in the Moment

Workshop Focus: As mortal creatures—creatures whose bodies will one day die—our time in these bodies is limited and therefore precious. Knowing this, we use the language of transaction to describe our relationship with time: we *pay* attention, and we *spend* time. Although God exists both in time and outside of it, dwelling in the present moment is how we best encounter God. This workshop invites participants to think of time—how we measure it and use it—in new ways and to practice releasing past and future to better inhabit the present moment.

This workshop is a good opportunity to ask people to practice silencing their phones, placing them out of sight, and to remove their wrist watches. Let all visible reminders of the passage of time be still.

Music Suggestions:

Peter Gabriel, "With This Love," track 16 on *Passion: Music for the Last Temptation of Christ*, Real World Studios, 1989. (arrival and check in)

Ulrich Schnauss, *Far Away Trains Passing By*, Domino, 2005. (opening meditation and flow)

MC Yogi, "Shanti (Peace Out)," track 13 on *Elephant Power*, White Swan, 2008. (closing Savasana)

Pranayama: Bee's breath, or the following prayer:

Instead of a pranayama we offer a one-line breath-prayer. We'll inhale on some words of the prayer and exhale on others. It's easiest if you say these words in your head instead of trying to speak them aloud. You'll inhale through your nose and exhale through your nose, exhaling with an almost audible sigh that sounds like wind in the trees. The inhale will be full, and the exhale will be as long as you can comfortably make it. Let's try it: inhale, filling the belly, ribs, and chest. Exhale slowly, letting the air release from the chest, ribs, and belly. Exhale it all out. Inhale. [*Repeat.*]

Continue this pattern of breath, and we'll overlay it with verse 10 from Psalm 46, a verse that helps us stop our thoughts from moving and instead stay in this present moment: "Be still and know that I am God." You can close your eyes if you like.

Inhale on "Be still"; long exhale on "and know that I am God." [*Repeat three times.*]

Continue your deep and controlled breathing. On this next set of three breaths we'll drop the word *God,* so inhale on "Be still"; long exhale on "and know that I am." [*Repeat three times.*]

On this next set we'll drop the words *I am*. Inhale on "Be still"; long exhale on "and know." [*Repeat three times.*]

And now just the words *Be still.* "Be" on the inhale; "still" on the exhale. [*Repeat three times.*]

And finally, the word *Be*: Inhale "Be"; exhale without words. Inhale "Be"; long, wordless exhale. Continue on your own. [*Repeat nine or twelve times.*]

Now return to normal breath. What are you feeling in this moment? Have your thoughts slowed down? What are you sensing in your body? Flutter open your eyes.

Yoga Teachings:

Think about a time in your life when you were completely unaware of time and time passing: Was it a project you were immersed in or a book that captivated you? Was it a walk and conversation with a dear friend that overflowed into something else you had scheduled?

These are moments in your life when you were pure awareness. No concept of time, not living in the past, not wishing for the future; just distinctly in the present moment: open-hearted, alive, and aware. In yoga this is considered "living in the flow"—a time when you are a part of everything around you and no separation exists. We forget ourselves and get lost in the flow of bliss. Unfortunately, these experiences don't seem to last very long or happen very often. Ram Dass said, "It is in these moments of your life that there is no longer separation. There is peace, harmony, tranquility, the joy of being part of the process. In these moments, the universe appears fresh; it is seen through innocent eyes. It all begins anew."[89]

In the world today, it can feel as if our moments of peace have been stolen from us. Our phones and devices bring news, social media posts, and work emails to us constantly, unless we make the conscious decision to silence them. Even in silence, the temptation to dream about better days ahead or return with

89. Ram Dass, "The Totality of the Moment," Love, Serve, Remember Foundation, accessed October 21, 2021, *https://www.ramdass.org/the-totality-of-the-moment/*.

nostalgia to times past is a strong one. How do we stay in today? With this breath and in this moment?

The answer is yoga. Yoga is more than asana. It is a way of living that helps us release the illusion that we are separate from others. The practice of the eight limbs of yoga—asana, breathwork, meditation, concentration, focus, enlightenment, how we treat ourselves, and how we treat others—leads us to a greater present moment awareness. This does not happen overnight, which is why it is called a *practice*—every day we take into account the teachings of yoga to make small changes in our lives: "The teachings allow us to shed our worries, self-doubt, judgements and regrets, and invite us into the present moment where we peacefully merge into the wholeness that is here for us Now."[90]

The ancient yogic text The Yoga Sutras of Patanjali is a guide for improving the mind so we can reach the highest states of momentary awareness: "It leads to a clearer perception and the ability to know the Self, which ultimately results in independence from suffering."[91] When our mind is less distracted and less irritated, there is a distinct calming and refining impact on our thoughts. We experience less anxiety and fear, and we connect with the flow of life and love. We know ourselves better, are more in control of our reactions, and make better choices. We feel more connected. In the wise words of Eckhart Tolle, "Realize deeply that the present moment is all you will ever have."[92]

Christian Teachings:

✝ In Christian theology there are two descriptions of time: chronos time and kairos time. Both come from ancient Greek. *Chronos* means a period or duration of time, or time that is measured. *Kairos* means a fitting season, a suitableness, a suitable place in the order of things, a season, an occasion, an opportunity. It resists measurement.

Chronos time has been called the time of the earth, of duration.[93] Chronos measures loss. Kairos time is the time of God, and sometimes it breaks into our chronological world: "Kairos contains *chronos* but is not bound by it. Chronos can never contain *kairos*, but it can be reshaped by it."[94] Chronos time measures

90. Dass, "The Totality of the Moment."

91. Kate Holcombe, "The Yoga Sutra: Your Guide to Living Every Moment," *Yoga Journal*, November 17, 2015, *https://www.yogajournal.com/yoga-101/yoga-sutra-guide-to-living-every-moment.*

92. "Eckhart Tolle," Goodreads, accessed October 21, 2021, *https://www.goodreads.com/quotes/259848-realize-deeply-that-the-present-moment-is-all-you-will.*

93. Barbara Cawthorne Crafton, *The Also Life* (New York: Morehouse Publishing, 2016), 14.

94. Crafton, *The Also Life*, 14.

loss, but in kairos nothing is lost. Past, present, and future are all contained within God.[95] In other words, because there is nowhere God is not, God is in *both* chronos time and kairos time. Even so, when we are able to encounter God it is likely because we have crossed from chronos time into kairos time. We cross into kairos time through meditation, through contemplative prayer, through yoga—any practice that helps us pay focused and sustained attention to the present moment and release our hold on the past and the future.

Modern physics has theorized about the elasticity of time, and I see this elasticity the most in kairos, or God's time. It helps make sense of the verse from the second letter of Peter, chapter 3, verse 8: "But do not ignore this one fact, beloved, that with the Lord one day is like a thousand years, and a thousand years are like one day."

✝ Italian physicist Carlo Rovelli says that the world consists not of things (objects) but happenings (events). In fact, "the world is a network of events."[96] "Things," he writes, "persist in time; events have a limited duration."[97] And yet even things have a shelf life. Consider the largest and hardest stone: over time—sometimes eons—it erodes under the assault of water and weather. Eventually, it becomes dust.

The apostle Peter, writing to persecuted Christians in Asia Minor, urged them to love deeply, from the heart, for that deep heart place was the only part of them that would endure. Everything else was impermanent. "All flesh is like grass [he said] and all its glory like the flower of grass. The grass withers, and the flower falls, but the word of the Lord endures forever" (1 Pet 1:24–25, quoting from Isa. 40:6–8).[98]

The impermanence of all things is one more bit of encouragement for living in the present. And if the world is a network of limited-duration events, that adds to the case for staying awake and aware in the present moment. To be fully alive is to be in the present moment.

✝ The pandemic altered our relationship with time. It changed the way we "dream forward" into the future because most of us had to confront futures that seemed far less certain than at any other time in our lives. The blessing hidden in the folds of this realization is that with the future dethroned as an object of focus, the way cleared for us to better practice living in the moment.

---

95. Crafton, *The Also Life*, 15.

96. Carlo Rovelli, *The Order of Time* (New York: Riverhead Books, 2018), 96.

97. Rovelli, *The Order of Time*, 98.

98. For additional scripture on flesh fading or withering like grass, see James 1 and Psalms 37 and 103.

In the sixth chapter of the Gospel of Matthew, Jesus offers an extended teaching on the futility of worrying about the future: "Therefore do not be anxious, saying, 'What shall we eat?' or 'What shall we drink?' or 'What shall we wear?' For the Gentiles seek after all these things, and your heavenly Father knows that you need them all. But seek first the kingdom of God and his righteousness, and all these things will be added to you" (Matt. 6:31–33 ESV). The implication is that those who do not know God waste time fretting about things that are already being provided for them. But if one seeks the kingdom of God—in other words, if one lives as a unitive thinker, oriented toward love and the pursuit of equity and justice—then one will discover that material needs have been addressed and filled.

Buddhist teacher Sharon Salzberg says that when we get swept up in desire for what could or should be (instead of accepting what is, in this moment) we become trapped in chronos or linear time. She writes that "it is as if before each breath ends, we are leaning forward to grasp at the next breath."[99] There is no peace in this, no stillness, no rest.

Henry David Thoreau, a nineteenth-century devotee of pranayama who was well versed in yogic texts like the Bhagavad Gita and the Upanishads, wrote, "You must live in the present, launch yourself on every wave, find your eternity in each moment. Fools stand on their island of opportunities and look toward another land. There is no other land; there is no other life but this."[100]

Suggested Asana Flows:

Warm-up

- Child's pose
- Tabletop
- Downward-facing dog
- Pyramid, right foot forward
- Forward fold—halfway lift—forward fold
- Hands over head pose
- Side bend right, side bend left
- Step back, right foot
- Pyramid post, left foot forward
- Plank

99. Salzberg, *Lovingkindness*, 55.

100. "April 24, 1859," This Date, from Henry David Thoreau's Journals, accessed October 21, 2021, *https://hdt.typepad.com/henrys_blog/2010/04/april-24-1859.html.*

- Baby cobra
- Downward-facing dog
- Child's pose

Flow

- Tabletop
- Cat-cow
- Bird dog, left leg back and right arm forward
- Gate pose, left leg, left side
- Side plank, right hand and knee down, left leg up
- Tabletop
- Cat-cow
- Bird dog, right leg back and left arm forward
- Gate pose, right leg, right side
- Side plank, left hand and knee down, right leg up
- Tabletop
- Downward-facing dog
- Warrior I, right foot forward
- Humble warrior
- Bound warrior III
- Warrior 1
- Extended side angle
- Reverse triangle
- Half moon balance on right leg, right arm down
- Release to forward fold
- Plank
- Child's pose
- Repeat opposite side

Cooldown

- Tabletop
- Lizard, right leg forward
- Twisted lizard, right side
- Locust

- ➢ Tabletop
- ➢ Lizard, left leg forward
- ➢ Twisted lizard, left side
- ➢ Lower onto belly
- ➢ Shoulder stretch through climbing tree frog, both sides
- ➢ Turn over onto back for bridge pose
- ➢ Waterfall
- ➢ Savasana

Closing Meditation: If you'd like to make this a walking meditation, you may, or you can sit or lie down on your mat. Whatever you choose, please make sure you are close enough to be able to hear. Whether you walk or put your body into stillness, do what promotes relaxation for you.

The text of this meditation comes from Ecclesiastes 3:1–8, which is well known beyond Judaism or Christianity. It's the passage that begins, "For everything there is a season and a time for every purpose under heaven." The passage consists of couplets, like "a time to be born and a time to die," a "time to mourn and a time to dance," and so on.

I'll read these verses once through, and then I'll read them again and unpack them a little. Listen for a word that elicits in you a strong reaction. See if you can become friends with that word.

For everything there is a season, and a time for every matter under heaven. In the Greek, every instance of the word *time* in this passage refers to kairos time, not chronos time, with one exception: this first verse. In it the words *kairos* and *chronos* are both used. It's another way of saying that God is in all things. All things are in God. Both measured time and suspended time are filled with God.

A time to be born, and a time to die. This can refer to the birth or death of any living creature. It can also refer to the birth or death of relationships, ideas, habits, and institutions. God is in all birthing and dying.

A time to plant, and a time to pluck up what is planted. Sometimes we get to harvest what we have never planted or tended. Other times we must plant and plant and plant again, never knowing if we shall see something bear fruit. God is in all harvesting and planting.

A time to kill, and a time to heal. Sometimes something harmful must be destroyed, and God is in the agonizing decision to do that. Sometimes something broken must be healed, and God is in the hard labor of reconciliation.

A time to break down, and a time to build up. God is equally in both the tearing down or the taking apart and also in the building up.

A time to weep, and a time to laugh. Be happy, our culture tells us. Keep going. Put one foot in front of the other, as if by determined walking we could successfully leave grief behind in the dust. But scripture says something different: both tears and laughter have their due time, and God is in both.

A time to mourn, and a time to dance. The wisdom is to make room in our lives for both grieving and celebrating and not to get locked into one as a way of avoiding the other.

A time to throw away stones, and a time to gather stones together. There is a time to trust the world and a time to be on guard against it. When Ecclesiastes was written, stones were weapons of war. There is a time to be carefree (throwing away stones) and a time to be watchful (gathering stones together). Again, the wisdom is to be able to release one state of being and move into the other, locked into neither.

A time to embrace, and a time to refrain from embracing. God is in both our enthusiasm—our embrace—as well as in our reticence—when we refrain from embracing. There is a time for both, depending on the situation. How sad to move through life always suspicious of everything and everyone, and how sad to move through life a trusting fool who lacks discernment.

A time to seek, and a time to lose. Recall the words of Sharon Salzberg, about the Buddhist philosophy of releasing or renouncing, and her caution about moving through life always leaning forward and seeking. Recall the words of Jesus: those who lose their lives for his sake will find them.

A time to keep, and a time to throw away. This can refer to the keeping and throwing away of experiences. How many hours of good sleep have we lost to fretting about something that happened that day? Someone hurt our feelings or we felt misunderstood. Can we keep the lesson we learned from this and throw the rest of the experience away? Jesus counseled his disciples to shake the dust off their sandals and move on if they encountered rejection. God is with us as we mine an experience for the lessons it can offer us, and God is also with us when we seek to release it.

A time to tear, and a time to sew. This verse echoes the verse about killing or destroying and healing or knitting together. Tearing speaks of separating. Sewing speaks of bringing together. There is a season for both, and both are filled with the presence of God.

A time to keep silence, and a time to speak. Christians talk a lot about speaking truth to power, yet sometimes there is wisdom in keeping silence. We often speak and regret it later, or say nothing and later think of the perfect retort. It takes humility to stop talking and listen. It takes courage to open your mouth and speak the words others perhaps fear to say. God attends both our humility and our courage.

A time to love, and a time to hate. The Greek φιλια [FIL-eh-oh] means kindness or affection. The Greek μισεω [mis-EH-oh] means to hate or detest, or it can also mean to regard with less affection, to love less. It isn't necessary to hear this verse as depicting two extremes or opposites of feeling. It's tempting to think that as people of faith we should be kind to everybody all the time and suppress all negative feelings. But anger and outrage at injustice are given us for a reason: to help keep us and the society in which we live pointed *toward* God instead of away. As with other couplets of emotion, the art is to not get stuck in hate, in a them-and-us mindset. Jesus got furious with people, but he didn't stay locked into that fury.

A time for war, and a time for peace. This last is a hard one to unpack, for Jesus had no explicit teachings about war. Why would that be? Ecclesiastes was written about three hundred years before the birth of Jesus, and the ancient world was perhaps more in turmoil. By the time of Jesus's birth, the Roman Empire was firmly established. Jews were oppressed, to be sure, but the world was more stable. Jesus certainly spoke about oppression because it was a reality in his lifetime, but he said little about war. This verse may simply indicate that in this imperfect world, God recognizes that there will be times of war and times of peace, and God will not abandon us in either.

There is no time, no season, no state of being where God is not. Rest in this assurance as we move into Savasana.

Workshop 9: Divine Incarnation–Yoga and Christianity Converse about the Sanctity of Human Flesh

Workshop Focus: Americans are exposed to thousands of advertisements every day. Many of those convey stereotypes about the human body—for example, portraying women as sexual objects or as housewives in pursuit of a germ-free home. Perpetual youth is held aloft as a universal goal, and we are urged to fight aging, as if it were an enemy instead of a natural biological process. The Victorian era infected us with a squeamishness and a prudishness about the human body from which Christianity has yet to fully recover. The advocacy of the LGBTQIA community and communities of color have shown us that our ideas about what is beautiful and natural are in dire need of a long-overdue, top-to-bottom overhaul.

The human body, in all its magnificent diversity, is an extraordinary creation. In addition to its dazzling biological systems, it is a dwelling place of God. This workshop seeks to help participants recover a sense of the marvelous beauty of the human body and to begin to embrace it (or more fully embrace it) as a temple of the divine.

Music Suggestions:

Peter Gabriel, "With This Love," track 16 on *Passion: Music for the Last Temptation of Christ*, Real World Studios, 1989. (arrival and check in)

Mark Ciaburri, *One*, Real Music, 2020. (opening meditation and flow)

Krishna Das, "Sri Argala Stotram," track 2 on *Kirtan Wallah*, Out, 2014. (closing Savasana)

Pranayama: Participants stand in mountain pose. Root down through the feet, relax the shoulders away from the ears, and close the eyes. *Viloma* breath (pausing breath) incorporates a conscious pause on inhales and exhales and brings awareness to bodily sensations. It can help release anxiety and stress. Inhale the arms up overhead and ask participants to pause, then exhale hands to the sides and ask participants to pause before inhaling again. Remind people they can skip the pause if it invokes feelings of nervousness or discomfort. Do this for three rounds, then have participants stand in mountain pose and begin an embodiment breath starting at the feet. An embodiment breath brings awareness to a body part by asking participants to inhale into it. Begin with the feet, and notice any sensations as the toes or feet pads ground into the mat. With each new inhale, slowly move up the body, from feet to calves, then knees, quads, hips, belly, and into the heart. Breathe through the shoulders, then down the arms into the fingertips, then up the arms into the neck. Breathe finally through the crown of the head. At each step, pause and invite awareness: How does my physical body feel? What are my thoughts and their feelings? This is also a great breath to return to in Savasana (supine mountain pose) at the end of the workshop.

Yoga Teachings:

The eight limbs of yoga, identified by Patanjali in his ancient book The Yoga Sutras, are all tied together by an invisible thread, called a sutra. The first two limbs, yamas and niyamas, are disciplines and observances. The next limb is asana, which is known as physical postures. We practice breath control, called *pranayama*. We withdraw our senses, called *pratyahara*. We focus our concentration, called *dharana*. We then meditate with a steady mind, called *dhyana*. Ultimately, we reach *samadhi*, the eighth limb. There we find complete union and harmony with our own Self—the divine within us—and with the divine beyond us. We find liberation from the confines of the physical body and from racing thoughts. Practicing the eight limbs in succession promises us freedom, bliss, and tranquility. These are divine attributes available to we who live in human bodies.

Our culture encourages us to seek these qualities not in the body but from outside sources using materialistic means. New cars promise us freedom, and if we acquire the right goods and experiences, we are promised bliss and tranquility. Even though our hearts tell us that purchasing an SUV does not grant us freedom and that beautiful clothes do not bestow happiness, the messages are alluring and powerful. Unfortunately, enlightenment cannot be so easily purchased.

There is a system to the lifestyle of yoga. Practicing our way through the eight limbs can move us toward enlightenment. Westernized yoga tends to focus foremost on the physical body, its anatomy, and the exercise benefits of the poses. Asana (the poses) is one of the first of the eight limbs undertaken, because it prepares the physical body for the next five limbs to follow. As B. K. S. Iyengar said, "The body is the temple of the soul. It can truly become so if it is kept healthy, clean, and pure through the practice of asana. Asanas act as bridges to unite the body with the mind, and the mind with the soul."[101]

Yoga has five branches. Jnana yoga emphasizes commitment to inquiry. Karma yoga is the commitment to one's life purpose or dharma. Bhakti yoga is the devotion to God and is often associated with prayer or chanting. Raja yoga emphasizes a commitment to introspection and contemplation. Lastly, hatha yoga is all about the physical body, building discipline through asana and pranayama to balance the mental and physical energies. Hatha yoga dates from the fifteenth century when a teacher named Svātmārāma set forth asanas (poses) and pranayama. He described the body as made of influences from the sun (*ha*) and the moon (*tha*) with exercises to do in order to balance these heavenly bodies within the physical body. Svātmārāma outlined an asana practice, dietary restrictions and suggestions, and moral and ethical guidelines for a yogi to keep his or her body balanced and healthy.

Yogic philosophy regards the body as the temple or sheath that protects the Self—the Atman, or the God within us. In Sanskrit the word for "body" is typically *deha* or *deham*; *de* for protect and *aham* for Self or Atman.

Although the body contains the divine, the body itself is not necessarily regarded as wholly divine, for it is subject to impurities, sickness, and death.

101. B. K. S. Iyengar, *Light on the Yoga Sutras of Patanjali* (St. Louis: The Aquarian Press, 1993), 29.

The Chandogya Upanishad tells a story that illustrates "the immortal and imperishable Self [the God within us] different from the perishable and physical body and its numerous organs." The aim in life is to liberate the soul from the body. This stands in contrast to Christian thought, which teaches that both body and soul bear the imprint of God and that, once resurrected, both will exist eternally. In the Episcopal burial liturgy, the opening words promise: "After my awaking he will raise me up and *in my body* I shall see God."[102]

Imperfect as the physical body may be, yogic philosophy still asserts that as the temple that protects the Atman, the God within, it should be accorded care and honor. In Vedic texts, the human body is variously described as a metaphor for the physical universe; as creation itself; as Nature; as a city, a chariot, a field, a vehicle, a battlefield, and a temple—to name a few.[103] Because yogic philosophy regards the body as perishable, it is sometimes thought to be a temporary construct or illusion. In some texts the body is seen as an obstacle, "responsible for the soul's bondage upon earth."[104] One purpose of the yamas and niyamas is to purify the body and thus diminish the power of bondage it represents. Yogic philosophy sees both the divine potential of the human body to be a vehicle of truth and liberation, and also its potential to be an agent of untruth, and a "means of delusion and ignorance."[105]

Christian Teachings:

✝ Mary, mother of Jesus, is called the *Theotokos*—the God-bearer. She carried in her womb the divine embodied in human flesh—the infant born into the ancient world as Jesus of Nazareth. Celtic spirituality maintains that *all* infants born are the divine embodied in human flesh. Theologian John Philip Newell says that since the fourth century, Celtic Christians have believed that when you look into the face of a newborn child you are looking into the face of God.[106] Such a perspective was promoted by the Welsh monk Pelagius, who would be denounced by Rome as a heretic. The church in Rome preferred the teaching of Pelagius's contemporary, Augustine of Hippo, who developed the doctrine we know as the doctrine of original sin.

---

102. *The Book of Common Prayer*, 491.

103. Jayaram V., "Human Body Symbolism in Hinduism," Hinduwebsite.com, accessed October 21, 2021, *https://www.hinduwebsite.com/symbolism/thebody.asp*.

104. Jayaram V., "Human Body Symbolism in Hinduism."

105. Jayaram V., "Human Body Symbolism in Hinduism."

106. John Philip Newell, lecture, April 20, 2018, St. Andrew's Episcopal Church, Denver, CO. In the lecture, Newell attributed this observation to the Welsh monk Pelagius (360–430 CE).

Pelagius versus Augustine: one man claimed we are born holy; the other man claimed we are born stained by sin. Because we are all descended from Adam, reasoned Augustine, we therefore all inherit his sinful nature. Newell says that for centuries Christians have obsessed over this doctrine, with the result that it has "haunted our souls."[107] Fortunately, there have always been those in the Christian tradition who push against the assumption of Augustine.

The fourteenth-century Christian mystic Julian of Norwich received a series of divine visions, and she wrote them all down. One of the many stunning revelations she offered was that we are not just made *by* God, but *of* God. We come from the very womb or essence of God. The love longings deep within us, that draw us toward one another and toward God, are deeper than the fears we harbor that tend to fragment us, separating us from one another and from God. What is deepest and most pure or authentic in us is not of some original sin, but of God.[108]

If there is an "original sin," says Newell, it is our forgetting that we are made in the image of God. Jesus came to remind us of our deepest identity, that which we had forgotten.[109]

✝ Psalm 139:13–16 describes a God who is inescapable, who exists everywhere. God companions us through life and death, beyond the grave, and is with us even before we are born. The psalmist says to God:

> For it was you who formed my inward parts;
>   you knit me together in my mother's womb.
> I praise you, for I am fearfully and wonderfully made.
>   Wonderful are your works;
> that I know very well.
>   My frame was not hidden from you,
> when I was being made in secret,
>   intricately woven in the depths of the earth.
> Your eyes beheld my unformed substance.
> In your book were written
>   all the days that were formed for me,
>   when none of them as yet existed.

We are fearfully made. The ancient Greek means we are reverently, awesomely, and honorably made. Don't you love the idea that God put you together, cell by

107. Newell, lecture.

108. These are Julian's teachings as shared by John Philip Newell in his April 20, 2018, lecture.

109. Newell, lecture.

cell, tissue by tissue, bone by bone, with reverence? For God, making you was an act of worship. *We are wonderfully made.* The Greek means we are distinguished, set apart, unique. Of all the glorious life forms with whom we share this earth, the human body is distinguished above them all.[110]

God does not merely form us out of nothing into something in the womb and then forget about us once we emerge into the world. God continues to shape and form us all the days of our lives. One might reasonably presume that divine work within us even continues after the death of our mortal bodies. The great French artist Paul Cézanne was said to create his masterpieces through a painstaking and endless process of sketches, studies, and adjustments. His creative process stood in sharp contrast to that of his friend and contemporary Pablo Picasso, who put paint to canvas as though a dam were about to burst inside of him. When it comes to the human person, the human body, consider God as a divine Cézanne—as involved and in love with the process of creating a masterpiece as with finishing and releasing it.[111]

✝ As Christianity took shape in the Greco-Roman world, it met Neoplatonism. In the Neoplatonic ordering of things, the spiritual is prioritized over the material or physical. The divine exists up above and humans, down below. This way of thinking led the ancients to assume that God could not possibly wish to descend from the divine realm into the muddy, messy, imperfect realm of the material world. The transcendent could not possibly wish to become immanent.

Amid this orderly paradigm, early Christians made the stunning claim that the transcendent divine had indeed desired to become immanent and had in fact done so in Jesus of Nazareth. If Neoplatonism was a serene pond, Christianity was a big boulder dropped into it from an impressive height. The ripples from that continue to push against our legs as we wade along the shore.

The Gospel of John (written 90–110 CE) put the stunning claim this way: "The Word became flesh and lived among us" (1:14a). Christianity began as an *enfleshed* spirituality, believing that God could be found in the human body and in the material world. Sadly, the church chose to devote its energy to explaining the problem of sin—how a perfect God could subsist inside an imperfect human container—and the implications of this extraordinary claim were not fully explored.

Except, that is, by the Christian mystics in every age who continued to ponder what it means to meet and find union with God in our bodies and in the

110. "Psalm 139," Bible Hub, accessed October 21, 2021, *https://biblehub.com/interlinear/psalms/139.htm.*

111. Malcolm Gladwell, "Late Bloomers," *New Yorker*, October 13, 2008, *https://www.newyorker.com/magazine/2008/10/20/late-bloomers-malcolm-gladwell.*

material world. They taught that "you don't have to deny the earth to embrace heaven. . . . You don't have to reject your body or your physical nature to embrace spirituality." Since in Jesus Christ God "became a human being, the nexus in all the universe where humanity meets divinity is right here, right now, in our mundane physical world."[112]

What are the implications of this for us? For starters, taking care of your body is not self-indulgent. Rather, it is taking care of a dwelling place of God.

Suggested Asana Flows:

Warm-up

- Mountain pose
- Side bend left, side bend right
- Chair pose, twist left, with right arm straight in front and left arm straight behind
- Hands over head pose
- Forward fold—halfway lift—forward fold
- Hands over head pose
- Chair pose; twist left, with right arm straight in front and left arm straight behind
- Hands over head pose
- Forward fold—halfway lift—forward fold
- Tabletop
- Cat-cow
- Child's pose

Flow

- Mountain pose
- Hands over head pose
- Goddess the arms
- Hands over head pose
- Forward fold
- Downward-facing dog
- Warrior I, right foot forward
- Humble warrior

112. Carl McColman, *The Big Book of Christian Mysticism* (Charlottesville, VA: Hampton Roads Publishing Co., 2010), 134.

- Bound warrior III
- Warrior I
- Extended side angle
- Triangle
- Pyramid
- Plank
- Lower down onto belly
- Baby cobra
- Downward-facing dog
- Repeat opposite side

Cooldown

- Easy seat
- Left leg bent, right leg straight; fold
- Right leg bent, left leg straight; fold
- Wide-legged seated fold
- Lie on back, pull right leg into chest, straight left leg
- Half happy baby, right leg
- Supine twist, both sides, crossing right leg to left side
- Come back to center
- Full happy baby
- Pull left leg into chest, straight right leg
- Half happy baby, left leg
- Supine twist, both sides, crossing left leg to right side
- Come back to center
- Full happy baby
- Savasana

Closing Meditation:

Option 1: Say while participants are resting in Savasana: "You are born into the physical body, the divine temple that houses and holds your spirit. In this resting pose, reconnect with your spirit through the *prana,* the life force that is your breath. Deeply inhale into the heart space of your being and awaken."

Bring participants out of Savasana and into a seated position. Place your hands at heart center in anjali mudra (prayer position), and take three deep breaths. Say to the participants, "As you stand at the threshold between yoga and your life beyond this class, take with you the knowledge that in you God delights in walking about in the world."

Option 2: John O'Donohue, a theologian of Celtic Christianity, writes that our bodies are a crowd of different members who work in harmony to make it possible for us to be in the world. He proposes we stop regarding our body and our soul as two different things. He further proposes we stop seeing our soul as hidden somewhere deep inside our body and says it's actually the reverse that's true. He writes, "Your body is in the soul, and the soul suffuses you completely. Therefore, all around you there is a secret and beautiful soul-light. This recognition suggests a new art of prayer: Close your eyes and relax into your body. Imagine a light all around you, the light of your soul. Then, with your breath, draw that light into your body and bring it with your breath through every area of your body." With your exhale, he says, release all the darkness or "inner charcoal residue." In this way, the light of the soul cleanses the body, bringing healing to the places that are tormented or neglected.[113]

Extras: With participant consent, snap a photograph of them—individually and as a group. Caption each photo of an individual: "I am a chosen dwelling place of the divine." Caption the group photo: "We are a chosen dwelling place of the divine." Email those to participants, and invite each person to print and place those photos near their home altar, yoga space, or meditation corner.

At an office supply store, buy an inkless fingerprint pad. On good-quality paper, create the image of a frame, blank inside. At the bottom print the words: *Uniquely made with reverence and delight.* Format two of these on a letter-sized sheet, and cut the sheet in half (so each is 5.5 inches by 8.5 inches). Or simply buy blank printable cards. Have one for each participant, and invite them to make a fingerprint (or a toe print) on the sheet or card as a take-home reminder of their intrinsic sacred nature.

Workshop 10: It's Golden–Yoga and Christianity Contemplate the Nourishing Necessity of Silence

Workshop Focus: The paradox of a workshop on silence is that by virtue of being a teaching and learning experience, it by necessity engages speaking, and speaking destroys silence. It's good to name that paradox before you get started, either as part of your advertising or as part of the welcome to the workshop, or

113. John O'Donohue, *Anam Cara: A Book of Celtic Wisdom* (New York: Harper Perennial, 2004), 49.

both. Silence is a vital nutrient for the soul, yet for many people, silence can be off-putting, even frightening. The goal of this workshop is to begin to explore silence in short segments. Use sparingly the teachings offered below. Instead of loading one workshop with numerous teachings, consider offering several workshops, each with no more than a teaching or two. However you elect to present the material, keep extemporaneous chatter to a minimum.

Acknowledge that many people resist silence because of what may arise for them in it, and use compassionate language to move participants from noise into silence. "I invite you into silence" implies you'll be there along with participants; they are not alone. "And now let silence befriend you, and let's explore being in relationship with it" implies silence can be a friendly presence. "I offer you the gift of a few moments of silence" reassures participants that the time of silence won't go on forever and that in today's relentlessly noisy world, silence is indeed a precious gift.

Music Suggestions: Consider music that is simple and sparse, and use it sparingly. This is not the time for an orchestra, band, or complex vocal harmonies, beautiful as they may be. Choose instrumental music with a slow and measured tempo that features a single instrument such as a cello, harmonium, recorder, or flute. If you choose vocal music, find a chant or song that does not demand the listener pay attention to the words. A soloist singing a Hildegard of Bingen piece is a good choice. Make sure the pieces chosen don't abruptly start or stop. Bring the volume up slowly, and fade out slowly when done.

Peter Gabriel, "With This Love," track 16 on *Passion: Music for the Last Temptation of Christ*, Real World Studios, 1989. (arrival and check in)

Voices of Ascension, *Voices of Angels: Music of Hildegard von Bingen*, Dios, 1997. (opening meditation and flow)

No music for Savasana—enjoy the silence.

Pranayama: *Nadi shodhana* (balance breath) or a basic breath that encourages awareness of the exhale and inhale.

Yoga Teachings:

Silence. What comes to mind when you think about this word? How does your body react when you think about being quiet? Silence. Some of us crave it; some of us fear it. In our neighborhoods and cities, silence can be difficult to find. Silence is often undervalued and is sometimes considered wasteful in our to-do-driven culture. In fact, silence is necessary and vital to calm our body, minds, and spirit to heal, listen within, and invite a creative process flow. You may find you have to schedule silence into your day to be assured of it. When we do manage to escape from noise, we face another obstacle: mind chatter. Is it truly quiet when our minds are still racing?

In yoga, mind chatter, or the "monkey mind," is first recognized in Sutra 1.2 as *chitta vritti*. The sutra states, "Yogah chitta vritti nirodahah" and is loosely translated as "Yoga is the cessation and restraint of the mind chatter."[114] Practicing the eight limbs of yoga helps us achieve ultimate conscious awareness (enlightenment, or Samadhi) of our thoughts and actions, and it helps us control our minds and reactions. However, we must first understand that our perceptions, thoughts, and feelings arise from experiences both present and past. Even childhood experiences leave their mark on the way we presently see the world. Further, we are bombarded with messaging, some we invite and some we do not (like advertisements). A tantric Buddhist monk and scholar named Saraha, who lived in India over a thousand years ago, wrote, "The whole world is tormented by words and there is no one who does without words. But only insofar as one is free from words, does one really understand words."[115] Such invasions into our consciousness make it challenging to discern reality and truth. It's on us to make opportunities to sit with our Self in silence and recall who we truly are in our heart of hearts. In the quiet and calming of the mind comes great reward.

Close your eyes and listen to your breath, listen to the noises around you, and observe what arises physically, mentally, and emotionally. [*Be still for at least five minutes in silence.*]

Bringing awareness back to your Self on the mat, and without self-judgment, note what came up for you. What arose for you may differ from what arose for others, but most of us share an initial discomfort with silence. Know that the eight limbs of yoga are intended to deepen our appreciation of silence as a welcomed friend. Practicing asanas or postures promotes physical flexibility and strength and can keep our minds off the grumbling of our aches and pains. Practicing pranayama moves and directs the life force prana to balance energy in the body and cleanse the lungs and cells with oxygen. Focusing on the breath allows the mind to settle and is a tool for meditation. Practicing pratyahara by withdrawing from the senses is a challenging but effective way to enter silence. Releasing the mind's focus on sensory input like smells, sounds, and tactile sensations eventually strips away everything but silence. The paradox is that in silence,

---

114. *The Yoga Sutras of Patanjali*, 3.

115. Ram Dass, *Paths to God: Living the Bhagavad Gita* (New York: Three Rivers Press, 2004), 262.

our senses may be heightened! When the mind slows down its processing, we can reach a level of *santosha*—contentment and full presence in the moment.

Physical sensations do have a role in a 2,500-year-old meditation practice called *vipassana*. The word means to see things as they really are. The meditation practice promises self-transformation through self-observation. It's been explained like this: "[Vipassana] focuses on the deep interconnection between mind and body, which can be experienced directly by disciplined attention to the physical sensations that form the life of the body, and that continuously interconnect and condition the life of the mind. It is this observation-based, self-exploratory journey to the common root of mind and body that dissolves mental impurity, resulting in a balanced mind full of love and compassion."[116] When we listen inward, we tune into a higher sense of self and realization that we are all one. Divine love is found in the silence, as are often the answers we seek. Swami Sivananda said, "Silence is the language of God. It is also the language of the heart."[117]

Yogic philosophy posits that there are four levels of speech and four corresponding levels of silence. The counterpart of spoken or verbalized speech is verbal silence. I know what I wish or intend to say, but I do not speak the words. Middle speech describes the words in my throat before they are spoken. The syntax of the sentence is formed, the inflection is prepared, the meaning I intend is in mind. Mental silence is when I inhibit those words from forming into syntax—I inhibit them from assembling themselves into an order in which they can be understood by you. Idea speech describes the words just before they reach middle speech, while they are still vague ideas. The corresponding level of silence is called *wooden silence*. In wooden silence, no ideas or images are formed, and the body and face are kept free of nonverbal expression. The fourth level of speech is called *supreme speech*. It has been described as "the unmanifest source from which all sounds, images, and ideas emerge. Abiding in this state is the true meditative silence."[118] The fourth and highest level of silence is nondual auspicious silence. It is full and complete silence, both verbal and mental.

In the Bhagavad Gita, Lord Krishna, the divine source of all being, says, "Among all the secrets, I am the Silence."[119] That verse can also be translated, "I am

116. "Vipassana Meditation," Dhamma.org, accessed October 21, 2021, *https://www.dhamma.org/en-US/about/vipassana*.

117. Dass, *Paths to God*, 263.

118. Annie Wilson, "Meditation on Silence: As Per Bhagavad Gita," Inner Light Publishers, accessed October 21, 2021, *https://www.inner-light-in.com/2012/07/meditation-on-silence-as-per-bhagavad-gita/*.

119. Wilson, "Meditation on Silence," translation of 10:38.

the silence of the unknown and the wisdom of the wise."[120] Contemporary Indian spiritual master Sri Amit Ray wrote, "Silence is the language of Om" and said that to feel the supreme love that is the divine, both external and internal silence are important. He notes that prayer need not be perfect or wordy. Silent remembering and pure intention are sufficient "to raise the heart to that Supreme Power."[121]

Christian Teachings:

✟ John O'Donohue, poet and scholar of Celtic spirituality, said,

> One of the great thresholds in reality is the threshold between sound and silence. All good sounds have silence near, behind, and within them. The first sound that every human hears is the sound of the mother's heartbeat in the dark lake water of the womb. This is the reason for our ancient resonance with the drum as a musical instrument. The sound of the drum brings us consolation because it brings us back to that time when we were at one with the mother's heartbeat. That was a time of complete belonging.[122]

If we belong to God, then what is the sound of God? Is it a heartbeat? Is it all sound or simply the sounds in nature? Is the sound of God silence, that state of the absence of noise that envelops all sound? The Persian poet Rumi said of silence, "In the silence between your heartbeat bides a summons. Do you hear it? Name it if you must, or leave it forever nameless, but why pretend it is not there?" He also said, "Silence is the root of everything. If you spiral into its void a hundred voices will thunder messages you long to hear."[123]

✟ From John O'Donohue, poet and scholar of Celtic spirituality: "To be genuinely spiritual is to have great respect for the possibilities and presence of silence. . . . It has been said that 'true listening is worship.'"[124] Rumi said, "This silence, this moment, every moment, if it's genuinely inside you, brings you what you need." And he encourages us to stop running away frantically from silence and to "move outside the tangle of fear-thinking." Let silence, he wrote, take you to the core of life.[125]

---

120. Bhagavad Gita, 188.

121. Wilson, "Meditation on Silence," quoting from "Om Chanting and Meditation" by Amit Ray.

122. O'Donohue, *Anam Cara*, 70.

123. "Rumi Quotes about Silence," AZ Quotes, accessed October 21, 2021, *https://www.azquotes.com/author/12768-Rumi/tag/silence.*

124. O'Donohue, *Anam Cara*, 71.

125. "Rumi Quotes about Silence."

If we understand the divine to be at the core of life—to *be* the core of life—then it follows that silence has the power to carry us home to God, in every moment of life.

✟ Silence is not only a powerful tool to use in solitude. In friendship with another person silence can hold the key to a profound expression of love. John O'Donohue, poet and scholar of Celtic spirituality, said,

> One of the tasks of true friendship is to listen compassionately and creatively to the hidden silences. Often secrets are not revealed in words, they lie concealed in the silence between the words or in the depth of what is unsayable between two people. In modern life there is an immense rush to expression. Sometimes the quality of what is expressed is superficial and immensely repetitive. A greater tolerance of silence is desirable, that fecund silence, which is the source of our most resonant language. The depth and substance of a friendship mirrors itself in the quality and shelter of the silence between two people.[126]

It's common to think of the disciples of Jesus as pupils, servants, or subordinates. But toward the end of John's Gospel (15:15), Jesus tells them he no longer thinks of them as his servants but as his friends. If that is so, reflect on this: the depth and substance of my friendship with Jesus (or with God) mirrors itself in the quality and shelter of the silence we share together.

✟ Cultivating regular times of silence is not only essential for our spiritual well-being. It is also vital for our physical and emotional health. Some common culprits of noise pollution include the steady noise of mass transit: aircraft taking off or landing, subways, elevated trains, busy highways. Living in proximity to these exposes us to the negative impacts of noise. Those impacts include higher levels of the stress hormones cortisol and adrenaline, higher blood pressure, increased risk of fatal heart attack, and slower development of learning and cognitive skills in children. Even hospitals have become generators of noise pollution. Over the last half-century, the rise in the number of machines and monitors in a patient room has led to a 20 percent increase in noise. This steady noise not only interrupts sleep at a time when the human body needs it most; it also can raise stress levels at an already stressful time.[127]

Researchers explain that "just as noise triggers a range of detrimental effects on the body's systems, silence can help heal those challenges. Studies

---

126. O'Donohue, *Anam Cara*, 112.

127. Amy Novotney, "Silence, Please," *American Psychological Association* 42, no. 7 (July/August 2011): 46, https://www.apa.org/monitor/2011/07-08/silence.

show that silence can actually stimulate new cell growth in the brain, improve memory, and release tension in the brain and body."[128] Low-income neighborhoods suffer disproportionately from exposure to incessant noise, so protecting our fellow human beings becomes an act of compassionate justice. What can be done? For starters, consider researching building codes in your town or city to learn if provision can be made to require the installation of sound-dampening materials during construction, especially in buildings adjacent to mass transit routes or hubs. Where those codes are lax, work to strengthen them. Where they are nonexistent, insist they be created. Advocacy on behalf of those who do not feel they have the power to speak out can be a holy act.

Suggested asana flows.

Warm-up

- ➢ Easy seat
- ➢ Head rolls
- ➢ Side bend left, side bend right
- ➢ Side twist left, side twist right
- ➢ Wide-legged forward fold
- ➢ Tabletop
- ➢ Cat-cow
- ➢ Stretch, left calf
- ➢ Gate pose, left side
- ➢ Tabletop
- ➢ Cat-cow
- ➢ Stretch, right calf
- ➢ Gate pose, right side
- ➢ Tabletop
- ➢ Thread the needle, both sides
- ➢ Child's pose

Flow

- ➢ Table top
- ➢ Downward-facing dog
- ➢ Warrior I, right foot forward

128. "The Benefits of Silence for Body and Mind," Kripalu Center for Yoga and Health, accessed October 21, 2021, https://kripalu.org/resources/benefits-silence-body-and-mind.

- Extended side angle
- Reverse extended side angle, right hand lifted
- Reverse triangle
- Five-pointed star
- Runner's lunge, left side
- Wide-legged forward fold
- Walk hands to right front foot; standing splits, balance on right leg
- Giva squats (three times)
- Return to top of mat
- Hands over head pose
- Forward fold—halfway lift—forward fold
- Hands over head pose
- Step right foot back into warrior I, left foot forward; repeat on that side

Cooldown

- Lie on back
- Extend right foot to ceiling and pull back for stretch
- Extend right foot to right side for stretch
- Supine twist, both sides
- Bridge pose to reset
- Extend left foot to ceiling and pull back for stretch
- Extend left foot to left side for stretch
- Supine twist, both sides, left leg to right side
- Bridge pose to reset
- Dip one knee at a time into center of mat with knees bent
- Straighten legs and arms; side crescent moon stretch to the right; side crescent moon stretch to the left
- Savasana

Closing Meditation: Francis Bacon was a seventeenth-century philosopher who is regarded as the father of the scientific method. He was also an Anglican with an abiding faith in God. He once said that "silence is the sleep that nourishes wisdom."[129] Savasana is a time of rest and integration for both body and mind. It asks of us our silence in order to do its good work. Silence is the sleep that nourishes wisdom.

---

129. *https://www.goodreads.com/quotes/8065296-silence-is-the-sleep-that-nourishes-wisdom.*

Move participants into Savasana, guiding them through relaxing one body part at a time, ending with the mind: Quiet and still the mind. Let it float in silence like a calm, safe, warm, dark pool of water.

Extras: Invite participants to journal about the noise in their lives. What for them is the noisiest time of the day? How do their personal habits (like playing music or watching television) contribute to the noise in the home? How noisy is the neighborhood in which they live? Ask participants to reflect on ways they can introduce more silence into their lives—even if that hard-won silence comes in increments as small as a few minutes.

SAMPLE SURVEY

Thank you for coming to [*title of workshop*]! Please help us serve you more fully by completing this survey and dropping it in the basket as you leave.

I came tonight because I desire more of a spiritual component in my yoga practice. ___ YES ___ NO

I learned something tonight about yogic philosophy. ___ YES ___ NO

I learned something tonight about Christian theology. ___ YES ___ NO

I felt spiritually fed by tonight's class. ___ YES ___ NO

I believe that what I learned tonight will help me off the mat. ___ YES ___ NO

I would come to other classes like this on different topics. ___ YES ___ NO

Any topics in particular you'd like us to cover in future classes?

____

Any other feedback you'd like for us to have?

____

Thanks for your feedback. May your path be blessed.

6

LEARNING FROM OTHER CHURCH YOGIS

The best teachers are those who show you where to look but don't tell you what to see.

—*author unknown*

LET IT BE KNOWN YOU'RE WRITING A BOOK on bringing yoga into the church, and you start to hear about colleagues who are already doing that. Speak to those colleagues, and they tell you about even more clergy and lay leaders who have welcomed a ministry of yoga into their worship spaces. I spoke at length with nine colleagues, lay and ordained—three who serve at cathedrals, five in parish ministry, and one a school chaplain—and that's just within the Episcopal Church.

The interviews I conducted likely represent just a small portion of those in the Episcopal Church who lead or welcome yoga in their worship spaces. Even so, despite the modest size of the data pool, common themes arose that are instructive for those wishing to start a ministry of yoga in their parishes.

I asked these yogis to tell me the story of how they came to practice yoga. For some of them, the story of becoming a yogi and the story of becoming a priest were braided together with God, the common strand. I asked them what it was that inspired them to begin a ministry of yoga at their churches. I asked them to identify the barriers or hurdles they encountered and how they addressed or overcame them.

They told me about the people they had in mind when they began their ministry and about the people who actually showed up to practice. We covered the practical questions of scheduling, finding suitable teachers, and whether to charge money for a class. Their yoga ministries took place in the worship space, except when there was compelling reason (for example, in one case a damaged and long-leaking church roof made the worship space temporarily unusable for any purpose—including worship) not to do so.

They told me about the content of their yoga classes—what worked and what they experimented with that invites further fine-tuning. They identified the gifts or fruits of this ministry, some of them unexpected. They shared with me their dreams about where, post-pandemic, they hoped this ministry could take their churches. I found them to be kindred spirits in far more than yoga and am indebted to them for their contributions to this book: the Rev. Caroline Kramer, rector, Episcopal Church of the Redeemer, Shelby, North Carolina; the Rev. Mark Genszler, rector, Christ Church Cobble Hill, Brooklyn, New York; the Rev. Ann Gillespie, senior associate rector and director of the Center for Wellness and Spirituality, Church of the Holy Comforter, Vienna, Virginia; Irene Beausoliel, Cathedral member and RYT (Registered Yoga Teacher), St. Mark's Cathedral, Seattle; Greg Bloch, director of communications, St. Mark's Cathedral, Seattle; the Rev. Diana V. Gustafson, assistant rector, St. Margaret's, Washington, DC; the Rev. Becky McDaniel, chaplain, St. Catherine's Episcopal School, Richmond, Virginia; the Very Rev. Dr. Michael Sniffen, dean, Cathedral of the Incarnation, Long Island, New York; the Rev. Jude Harmon, Canon for Innovative Ministries, Grace Cathedral, San Francisco; and the Rev. Jonathan Thomas, corector, St. Paul's, Peoria, Illinois.

This chapter offers twelve insights for the priest or lay leader seeking to begin a ministry of yoga in the church. Each insight is supported by portions of the stories my colleagues so generously shared. Taken together, these insights provide wise counsel that can help ensure the success of a yoga ministry and its contribution to the thriving of a parish.

1. Leaders who welcome yoga are already unapologetically outward-facing in their ministry focus.

This is not to imply they subordinate or dismiss the importance of worship, the spiritual formation of their members, or pastoral care. It means, rather, they are always alert to ways their ministries can serve as bridges to the greater community, drawing people in. They encourage their existing members to look and act beyond the comfortable and familiar bounds of the parish. It's been said that "outreach is what happens when you leave the baptismal font."[1] The clergy and lay leaders I interviewed are teaching and modeling this very conviction to their congregations.

1. The Rev. Dr. Patricia Lyons, keynote address, October 4, 2019, Episcopal Diocese of Colorado annual convention.

The economic decline of a community inevitably affects the churches in that community and can be a natural catalyst for a church to look beyond its doors. Mark Genszler served a couple of parishes in this situation. At one his mission was to convince his parishioners that engagement with the community and experimentation in ministry could promote stability. At another, he arrived to find a parish in exile from its worship space due to structural damage sustained in a lightning strike. Worship services had to be relocated to the parish hall. Neither parishioners nor the community wanted to close the historic urban church, but something had to be done to arrest its decline. While they were figuring out how to make the repairs (a complex and costly process that ended up taking years), Mark offered parish hall space to two local charitable nonprofits, which meant that worship and charitable aid were happening in the same physical space.

One, a mutual aid society, used the space to store air conditioners and cartons of diapers for people in need. The other, a flower rescue group, used the space to turn the cast-off flowers they had salvaged from retailers into floral arrangements to brighten the rooms of the elderly and the poor. Mark sees his small parish membership as a eucharistic community that formed the heart or "strong center" of the church, and the community groups with whom they partnered as expressions of the parish's permeable boundaries and open doors. A community member read about a blood drive that needed a place to operate, and, knowing of the church's open doors, approached Mark, who said yes. Mark notes the embodied theology of people giving blood in the same space in which the Eucharist is celebrated. "Let those with ears," he smiles, "hear."

Mark calls the community groups who use Christ Church's worship space *congregations* and was gratified when he saw members of each of those congregations show up for church on Christmas Eve. Perhaps if sorting flowers or hauling air conditioners is introduced and promoted as an opportunity to encounter the divine, it is, in its way, a valid act of worship. Bringing yoga into the worship space after the pandemic will be simply a continuation of this outward-looking theology.

Born and raised in England, Caroline Kramer is quite familiar with the Fresh Expressions movement, an outward-looking initiative that was started in 2004 by the Church of England and the British Methodist Church. Fresh Expressions recognizes the sacred character and potential of non-Eucharistic gatherings that may take place beyond the constraints of front-facing pews and an altar, and it cultivates "new kinds of church alongside existing congregations to more effectively engage our growing post-Christian society."[2]

2. "About," Fresh Expressions, accessed October 21, 2021, *https://freshexpressionsus.org/about/*.

Each Fresh Expression gathering is highly contextual and brings Christian teachings and community to those who might not yet have experienced it. In these gatherings, church members do not seek solely to draw people into an existing church building. Instead, they go to where others gather. Although this is different from the ministry of inviting yoga into a church worship space, it shares one important thing in common with yoga in the church: a willingness to expand the definition of *church* and *worship*.

Like many churches affected by crumbling local economies, Caroline's parish had been treading water for some time before her arrival. The church was located in a low-income neighborhood, and Caroline wanted to reach the church's neighbors with yoga, offering them something widely regarded as the exclusive property of "white, skinny, middle-class girls with expensive coffees."[3] She wanted to break this stereotype about yoga and offer without fee something many people couldn't otherwise afford. She wanted to teach her neighbors to love themselves as they are and saw the potential of yoga to further that goal. The pandemic paused the development of this ministry but only for a time. Caroline had tilled the ground by teaching weekly art classes to the neighborhood children. Yoga will be a natural outgrowth of that relationship she has built with her neighbors. If yoga can be thought of as a kind of body-liturgy, Caroline is using liturgy as mission.

She makes an important distinction, however: yoga will not be a means to preserve the institution by increasing the number of people in the pews on a Sunday morning. In other words, yoga is not intended to be a life ring tossed to a parish just keeping its head above the waves. Indeed, yoga in the worship space might even *challenge* the institution. For her it is about expanding the definitions of *church* and *worship* and seeing where the Spirit leads. This calls to mind Jesus's teaching that we must be willing to lose our lives to find them.

In contrast with parish churches that identify with a specific neighborhood or community, cathedrals are meant to serve the people of an entire diocese, and most cathedrals also try to live their call to be a sacred gathering place for people who may not affiliate as Episcopalian or even Christian. Cathedrals are by design outward-looking. Steve Thomason, dean of St. Mark's Cathedral in Seattle, threw the influence of his office behind Cathedral Yoga from the beginning, personally promoting it and inviting people to call him if they had questions. When bringing a new ministry into a church, a clergy leader's personal advocacy can lend the ministry legitimacy. If a leader is curious and excited, it encourages the people to be so as well.

---

3. The Rev. Caroline Kramer, interview with author, Zoom, January 20, 2021.

The unique and phased history of how the present St. Mark's worship space came to be made doing yoga there something of a nonissue. No one generation designed the space or funded it. Rather, it has elements from many different decades, so the sense of ownership feels more open than narrow. The nave and chancel are treated reverently, as sacred space, but the space itself is not worshiped. There's a history of radically reimagining the space or the activities taking place therein. The worship space has hosted canvas labyrinth installations, fundraising dinners, and theatrical and film presentations (including a screening of *The Hunchback of Notre Dame*, complete with live organ accompaniment).

Perhaps the best known alternative use of St. Mark's worship space is their service of Choral Compline, a beloved Sunday night offering of the cathedral since 1956. From the beginning, the service attracted community members who were otherwise not churchgoers, and it welcomed (and has always welcomed) those who preferred to lie on the floor instead of sit in the pews. The use of the whole body in worship is thus part of St. Mark's DNA.

At St. Paul's in Peoria, Illinois, the church (a former cathedral) stewards an enormous space: 54,000 square feet. The worship space is open, on one level, with an altar in the center between two banks of pews that face each other. It naturally lends itself to different expressions of worship. The church has sixteen classrooms that once housed a Montessori school.

When co-rectors (and spouses) Jonathan Thomas and Jenny Replogle were called to St. Paul's, they encountered an aging congregation in a working-class neighborhood—a congregation whose members recalled fondly their days as a cathedral and now thought of themselves as "just a parish." Jonathan helped them see that as a parish, they had a new calling: to serve the geographic area in which they were located. To do this they needed to forge better connections with the community.

Jonathan told the parish that they needed to steward their massive space. He challenged them to consider that any quest for survival was equivalent to clinging to their old ways. He pointed out that survival is not a Christian value. He challenged them to define what exactly they meant when they called St. Paul's "our" church. Did "our" mean "we own this"? Or did "our" mean "we belong to this"? He taught that there's a world of difference between the two, and the latter was what he hoped his members would embrace. The church website underscores this, with the tagline "You belong at St. Paul's." This may seem like a mere nuance of semantic, but the difference in ecclesiology is profound. Only with the latter attitude can a congregation truly welcome in the community.

Having established a vision of how the church might go forward, Jonathan and the parish looked for ministry partners in the community. They invited artists to fill the old classrooms and created an art colony. They found a connection with Soul Side Healing Arts, a yoga studio that also specialized in supporting those healing from trauma. Straddling the line between the business district of Peoria and the poorest zip code in all of Illinois, Soul Side was committed to making yoga accessible for people who couldn't afford it. Their pay-as-you-can policy synced well with St. Paul's, who was not out to make a profit but to engage with the surrounding community.

Three and a half years into their ministry at St. Paul's, Jonathan and Jenny invited Soul Side to offer a four-session introductory series on yoga and meditation. Perhaps because Jonathan had already cast a vision for their church that included community engagement, parishioners were supportive of the idea of yoga in the worship space. In the last six years, about half the parish membership is new and includes LGBTQIA couples and young families. Because of years of shifting diocesan dynamics and changing demographics, it is now the only Episcopal church in a forty-five-mile radius.

2. Leaders who welcome yoga into their churches are entrepreneurial and strategic.

None of the clergy welcoming yoga into the church worship space attempted to bring yoga into the church out of the blue or capriciously. All of them identified and built on some existing ministerial success in the parish.

Before Mark Genszler came to St. Francis, a large organic garden had been planted on the church's one-acre grounds as a way for the parish to reinvigorate engagement with the surrounding community. Mark calls the garden a low threshold for people to step over into the life of the church. As he got to know the folks, from both church and community, who worked in the garden, he sensed a yearning among them for something more. One day in the garden, a young mom from the community approached him and asked if he'd permit a yoga class in the parish hall. It would be geared to mothers and their young children, many of whom were homeschoolers. Philosophically, it was an easy yes, because a number of community groups already used the parish hall. While most of them paid something in consideration, they did so on a sliding scale. The yoga class charged enough to compensate the teacher and make a small donation to the church.

To have so many groups using the parish hall says good things about a church. The parish hall was already scheduled on the day that suited the organizers, a problem that Mark simply regarded as an opportunity, so he got creative. "Why don't you hold the class in the worship space?" he asked. The young mom was surprised. Mark sought to intentionally blur the bounds between church and community, between sacred and secular, seeking to make those bounds permeable.

This blurring of boundaries is life-giving and is supported by science—in particular, cellular biology: "The membrane [of a cell] is semipermeable, letting in energy and matter in continual exchanges with its environment. Without that permeability, nothing new could be created, and, like all closed systems, the young life form would quickly wear down and die. . . . Life cannot be sustained when the boundary becomes rigid."[4] Too much permeability can be as threatening as too little. Organisms flourish when there is a balance. What an apt metaphor for a faith community. Most of our churches do not suffer from too much permeability. We suffer from not enough.

At St. Francis, the nave had already been reconfigured at the suggestion of the bishop's office, to better reflect that the congregation was a blending of two small parishes (one building closing, St. Francis remaining open) and that all things—including the worship space—were being made new. The reconfiguration had removed some pews, so the space could easily accommodate yoga mats.

The yoga class ran for a time until some of its founding families moved away. Like many ministries, the family yoga program had a life cycle, and Mark allowed that cycle to play itself out and then built on that ministry's success: after the family yoga program ended, Mark secured a grant to work with neighborhood children in the church garden, and he incorporated yoga into that ministry. Expanding the definition of *sacred*, he taught that Christ is everywhere. He was especially gratified to be able to teach the children the nuances of silence—that it is not the absence of sound but rather filled with presence and that that presence is God. God is thus as near to us as our own breath. This is, of course, a key theme in yogic philosophy.

The ministry of Michael Sniffen offers an example of how opportunity can even be found buried in catastrophe. Before serving as dean of the Cathedral of the Incarnation (Diocese of Long Island), he was the rector of St. Luke and St. Matthew in Brooklyn, a dynamic congregation with a largely West Indian demographic. It was a small congregation in a big building with a good deal of deferred maintenance. The worship space was stunning, designed for 1,800 people, and had Tiffany windows. Michael and the congregation were looking for ways to bring the community into the space.

---

4. Margaret J. Wheatley, *Who Do We Choose to Be? Facing Reality, Claiming Leadership, Restoring Sanity* (Oakland, CA: Berrett-Koehler Publishers, 2017), 64–65.

As part of their effort to bring the community in, they invited a Juilliard choreographer to be an artist in residence. The parish hall was in essence a nineteenth-century dance hall—with a leaky roof. They got a grant to repair and upgrade the space as a dance studio. Part of the arrangement was that the choreographer would offer free dance classes to neighborhood children. They also taught yoga.

In October 2012, Hurricane Sandy ravished the area. The church was one of the founders of Occupy Sandy, the relief effort organized to help victims of Hurricane Sandy, and the sanctuary was used for hurricane relief work. This meant the congregation worshiped in the parish hall. Following this, an arsonist set the building on fire, and the congregation's temporary exile to the parish hall was extended. What this now meant was that dancers, relief meals, yoga, and worship all took place in the same space. Without pews defining it, the space welcomed different uses. People felt freer to move about it.

Michael regards a clergy leader as a "leader-follower": a faith community leader committed to following the Holy Spirit as a kind of celestial navigator. He observed that a leader must be improvisational, listening, watching, and continually asking, "How do we find a way to say yes to God?" Sometimes saying yes means looking for the openings the Spirit places in front of us. One proverb advises, "The way will open before you." The Quakers have a similar teaching: "Have faith, and the way will open." I sometimes wonder how often the Spirit opens the way for us and we miss it because we're otherwise engaged.

Caroline Kramer practiced paying attention to these openings and used them to build a yoga ministry in her church. In her second year as rector, a donor stepped forward to pay for twenty yoga mats and props, which was a powerful affirmation. Caroline put down temporary gym pad flooring over the stone floors of the worship space, and mats went on top of that. With fixed pews and stone floors, the worship space was not ideal for yoga, but they could fit twenty mats in it. She drew on the one yoga teacher already a member of the parish and another one from the community who was interested. She used the resources the Spirit offered her. To do so is both faithful and entrepreneurial.

3. Leaders who welcome yoga into their churches know first-hand what it can do for the body and the soul.

They have worked out for themselves a personal theology of yoga in the church and can articulate why yoga in a worship space is "meet and right so to do."

Diana Gustafson began practicing yoga fifteen years ago. She had been a runner, but when she hurt her back, her sister suggested she try yoga. Diana did, and her back stopped hurting. She found she loved the sense of community and the spiritual experience yoga offered. She found yoga offered a community where people don't just speak about love—they practice it. In a yoga community the practitioner focuses on a journey into the self, and yet often when people roll up their mats at the end of a class, it's plain that their focus is less about the self and more about the other.

Caroline Kramer has practiced for less than a decade and was motivated to begin by a desire to sustain joint mobility, a common desire among practitioners. Like many people, she was initially resistant to starting a practice because of her preconceptions about yoga, but she was urged by her three children to try it. At first she went in part to appease them. She found that she fell out of some of the asanas but also could manage to achieve others thanks to her natural flexibility. That encouraged her to keep going. She did her 200-hour yoga teacher training, which her vestry supported by paying half the cost. She went on to study for her 300-hour teacher training certification.

Some clergy were introduced to yoga as part of a background in theater. Mark Genszler, who's practiced on and off for twenty years, reflects on his childhood participation in community theater and recognizes that the theater director engaged yoga—although not by name—as a warm-up routine before rehearsals or classes and even offered a kind of Savasana.

Ann Gillespie was a television and film actress and was introduced to yoga in acting school in the late 1970s. The practice of yoga helped teach her to be comfortable in her own body and realize her own interior beauty, an important thing in an industry that prizes external appearances. Later, yoga stabilized Ann through having babies and then young children in the house. She trained in Santa Barbara in 1994 and began teaching. Teaching yoga honed her skills at reading a room, so in that way it supported both her acting career and, later, her vocation as one leading worship.

Others discovered yoga in college. Michael Sniffen took a course on yoga as part of his major in religion and minor in theater and dance. The course opened him to the spiritual growth possibilities of yoga beyond its usefulness as an exercise program. Becky McDaniel majored in religion with a minor in Tibetan Buddhism. Her first encounter with yoga was not with asanas but with dhyana, the meditation limb. She began practicing yoga after college, while she was teaching in a Title 1 school, serving low-income or low-achieving students. It was a challenging experience, and yoga helped her mediate the stress. Irene Beausoliel earned a BFA in dance and discovered yoga as part of that major. It helped her manage pain from injuries and allowed her to better bring her spiritual self into dancing. With this background she is able to model and teach what embodied worship can look like.

Still others, like Greg Bloch and Jonathan Thomas, had only a short or a sporadic background in yoga before they brought it into their churches. Despite their varying degrees of prior involvement, all those interviewed had sufficient introduction to yoga to know what it was they were inviting into the worship space. Those considering starting a church yoga ministry can benefit from having at least a year of personal experience with it.

4. Leaders who welcome yoga into their churches know it can be a gentle doorway into the life of the church, seeing its potential to remove barriers to church membership even while membership growth is not a stated or implicit objective.

All those I interviewed are content to let the Holy Spirit do her work. As Paul said in his first letter to the Christians at Corinth, God makes each of us servants through whom others come to believe (3:5b–7). We plant, others water, and God gives the growth. The clergy who welcome yoga practitioners into their churches do so with humility and gentleness. They know intuitively that many people who venture into a church to practice yoga have felt judged, alienated, or wounded by the church experiences of their past. As a result, those who offer yoga in the church are careful to avoid proselytizing, and they demonstrate a deep respect for wherever people happen to be on their faith journeys—even if where they are is a place of distrust of the Christian institution.

At St. Francis, Mark Genszler saw the surrounding area as one with a preponderance of cars and strip malls, and yet his small parish was not necessarily a reflection of that. In some respects, the parish was a draw for local folks who were inclined toward homeschooling and organic gardening. When he said yes to the young mom who wanted the church to host yoga classes for parents and their children, he hoped she would be a draw for young families from the community. And she was. About a dozen parents and their children came from the community several times a month. There were a few young families in the parish at the time, and it would be understandable if Mark saw the yoga ministry as a pipeline into the church. But he didn't. Mark didn't expect or try to make the yoga attendees into instant St. Francis members. Endued with the gift of patience, he let them lead the way. Some families sought him out for pastoral counseling. Some began to volunteer in the parish garden. A few showed up on Sundays. Some came for Christmas or Easter services. He planted, let others water, and God give the growth.

Caroline Kramer's degree was based on a study of liturgy as mission. At one large church where she served on staff, her ministry focus was worship and evangelism. She observes that spiritual but not religious (SBNR) folks are typically a favorite target for evangelism efforts, yet her academic study and her work in evangelism suggested that any direct attempt to engage them as potential church members would be clumsy at best and could do more harm than good. She understood that yoga practitioners (who as a group are certainly not synonymous with the SBNR but include a good number of them) and Christians are pointing at the same thing, pursuing the same general goal of union with a universal spirit beyond themselves; they're just using different language. That realization for her opened up a sense of possibility as to how the church might engage more humbly with those who are spiritually curious.

Jude Harmon at Grace Cathedral in San Francisco helped oversee a survey of their yoga participants and learned that 65 percent are aged forty or under, 35 percent are over age forty, and the majority come from the surrounding community. Jude estimated that of 800 souls who practice yoga in the cathedral, the number who were cathedral members was less than fifty. Even those attendees who are not cathedral members tend to think of yoga at Grace as "their church." Jude sees evidence of healing as people approach him with tears in their eyes. Others approach him for pastoral consolation over an eviction or job loss. Over the years the leadership philosophy has shifted from turning yoga attendees into Sunday morning worship service attendees to instead broadening the definition of what it means to be a cathedral member.

Jonathan Thomas pointed out that a church can lower the threshold to participation in the life of the parish in ways as small and practical as scheduling. Sometimes, the thoughtful or strategic scheduling of a yoga class can invite participants to explore further. At St. Paul's in Peoria Yoga in the Church is held on Sunday afternoons at 3:30 p.m. It concludes just as preparations are underway for a 5:00 p.m. contemplative service of Holy Eucharist. It is a natural flow from one event to the next, and occasionally a yogi will attend Mass. Greg Bloch and Irene Beausoliel note that Seattle abounds in yoga studios, classes, and workshops. What sets St. Mark's Cathedral Yoga apart (aside from being free of charge) is that it is designed to be a contemplative experience. People who find themselves drawn to it can take an easy next step and try out Choral Compline or other services in the Daily Office.

At the Cathedral of the Incarnation, Michael Sniffen creates easy doorways by making Yoga in the Cathedral free of charge, although a freewill offering is taken. Michael doesn't teach, but he generally participates. When inside, the space is candlelit, because there is something about candles that gentles any setting. The practice itself is inclusive of all abilities; it is not rigorous. Michael generally sets the class context but in a way that isn't didactic, for he believes an economy of words best sets the desired class tone. He might share what the cathedral is doing, like, "This week the cathedral begins the season of Lent." He might say a brief word or two about what Lent means to Christians and then pose a wondering question to the class participants. He believes that the signs and symbols of Christianity that surround the yogis in the worship space often speak more eloquently than can any person. He does everything he can to create an embodied worship experience that puts participants at ease. Michael understands that the ministry of all cathedrals is to be places of low-barrier entry for the community, and I applaud his commitment to "not just opening the doors to the community but tearing them off their hinges."[5] What kind of a denominational renaissance might we all enjoy if everyone shared this same commitment?

5. Leaders who welcome yoga into their church understand that their classes will be populated primarily by beginners.

All interviewees acknowledged the sacred trust participants placed in them to provide a safe and nonjudgmental yoga experience. Wanting to welcome those who wished to try out yoga before committing to buying all the gear, Jonathan Thomas encouraged St. Paul's to purchase twenty yoga mats to lower the barrier to participation for first-timers.

At St. Mark's, Cathedral Yoga attracts a wide range of ages, races, gender identities, and ability levels. People have diverse reasons for attending. People recovering from injury have found Cathedral Yoga safe and restorative. The classes appeal to beginners looking for a safe, accepting, accessible practice. Those with physical impediments have found Cathedral Yoga welcoming and doable. Cathedral members seem to be in the minority of attendees, perhaps because the yoga classes are scheduled early on a Sunday evening and many of those who attend Sunday morning worship have already left the city and gone home for the day. When the University of Washington is in session, a number of students attend, because Cathedral Yoga is free and easily accessible by bus or walk from campus.

Caroline Kramer offered yoga every other week and noted most of her attendees were parishioners of widely varying ability levels. She pointed out that timid first-timers or older practitioners might reasonably assume that yoga

5. The Very Rev. Michael Sniffen, interview with author, Zoom, February 16, 2021.

in their church would, by virtue of being *in their church*, be more welcoming and feel safer than what they might expect in a studio. This is an important assumption for those wanting to develop a ministry of yoga in the church to keep in mind.

Diana Gustafson tends to create more rigorous classes and acknowledges that to some degree this limits who will come. Even so, she takes great care to offer whatever asana modifications are needed, depending on the makeup of the attendees. She's had pew-sitters, folks in wheelchairs, and athletes all in the same class. All registered yoga teachers are schooled in how to modify asanas according to the abilities of the people who show up. Even so, yoga studio classes are usually categorized by ability and advertised accordingly. In general, at a yoga studio students tend to self-select the level of difficulty that works for them. Yoga in the church casts a much wider net, and someone teaching in a worship space needs to be prepared to teach to all levels simultaneously.

6. Leaders who welcome yoga into their churches may see the ancillary value yoga can offer as a tool for healing trauma, racial reconciliation, or building equal opportunities for underserved communities.

When Michael Sniffen started yoga at the Cathedral of the Incarnation, the yogis in the cathedral community were not all instant fans of the idea, yet within six months they were committed to the new ministry. They experienced and saw the potential of Yoga in the Cathedral to heal religious trauma. They realized they could come to class as whole and integrated persons (who, by virtue of being human, were broken in many ways) and not as "church people" (intent on putting on their best and most pious faces for God). I've heard Episcopalians joke that our churches are the place to see and be seen on a Sunday morning, and this joke usually elicits laughter. But sometimes humor edges uncomfortably close to the truth—that many of us "love to stand and pray in the synagogues and at the street corners, so that they may be seen by others" (Matt. 6:5). Maybe we think we can hide our real brokenness from God, or at least from our fellow worshipers. It's harder to do that in yoga.

Jonathan Thomas doesn't do much, if any, theological teaching in the yoga classes at St. Paul's. But he maintains that one should not downplay the power of the space itself. Like other clergy who have invited yoga into their worship spaces, he notes how healing it is for people who have felt wounded by a religious institution to be practicing yoga in the worship space of a Christian church. Doing so lets them see that the church cares about them as a total or holistic human being. "The Church *should* care about the physical health of its members," says Jonathan, "but all too often that aspect of health gets overlooked." We focus on the spiritual health of our members and forget that God chooses to live in our human, physical flesh, so we ought to take better care of it.

In her role as director of the Center for Wellness and Spirituality at Church of the Holy Comforter in Vienna, Virginia, Ann Gillespie hopes the Center will be a portal into the life of the church, a place where people can create a spiritual identity larger than themselves and become agents of healing and transformation in the world. One way that is already beginning is the addition of yoga and body awareness to the parish's racial reconciliation work. Inspired by the book *My Grandmother's Hands: Racialized Trauma and the Pathway to Mending Our Hearts and Bodies* by Resmaa Menakem, Ann added a body component to the Episcopal Church's Sacred Ground racial reconciliation program. I believe she is at the forefront of such work.

7. Leaders who welcome yoga into their churches see the benefit of helping their congregations develop a faith that lives in bodies and hearts as well as minds.

I heard a convention speaker say, "Each human being is a living creche for the God who said, 'I will come and rest in human flesh.' Not just to visit it but to come and dwell in it and to suffer in it."[6] My body is the manger where God waits to be born in the world. Your body is too. Every human body is a manger for the waiting God.

Animals of all kinds prepare a manger for their young waiting to be born. Birds build nests, dogs rearrange the towels laid in whelping boxes, turtles might scoop a depression in the sand. How do we humans prepare the "living creche" of our bodily selves for the waiting God? I'm not sure there's a ready answer to that question, because centuries of Neoplatonic dualism have laid down their influence on us like layers of dust. In general, the church has done a poor job of teaching the sanctity of the human body as a birthing place and dwelling place for God. Across Christianity, bodily sanctity has been sloppily shorthanded to mean "no pleasure, no fun, no sex." No wonder we find other things to teach and preach about.

That we might actually encounter God *in our bodies* is a novel idea for many of us. Ann Gillespie is doing exciting work on this front. While she was in

6. The Rev. Dr. Patricia Lyons, keynote address, October 4, 2019, Episcopal Diocese of Colorado annual convention.

seminary, she did an eight-week yoga series called "Finding God in Your Body." This led her to offer similar series and retreats at parish churches and to develop her own unique brand of yoga in church. As a class theme she might focus on a particular body part, open with meditation, and maintain a gentle background monologue of plain-language theology to guide people to notice where they're experiencing God in their bodies at that moment during the class. She uses asanas to talk about God, life, and worship. She has taken apart the poses of worship—standing, sitting, kneeling—and examined how each helps the body encounter the divine. Doing yoga in the church gives her a bigger vocabulary to talk about God than one would have in a yoga studio.

Interviewed during the pandemic, Becky McDaniel stated that what she misses is the Holy Eucharist. She finds deep parallels between the Eucharist and a yoga class. One theme of the Eucharist is that of healing through the act of being broken—the broken bread, the broken body (Christ's, ours, the church's). The sacrament asks of us our bodily (we kneel) and emotional (our open hearts) vulnerability. A yoga room is likewise a place and experience that invites us to be vulnerable to our emotions, so that broken open, we might begin to heal. Becky finds that during Savasana, placing a cool cloth on the forehead of a yogi can be a sacramental act, with ties to Jesus washing feet in the thirteenth chapter of John.

Children come perhaps pre-equipped to find God in their bodies, but we seem to train that out of them. Part of raising a child who is a good citizen of the world is teaching them to build a considerate awareness of the needs of people beyond themselves. That's a good and necessary thing, yet I wonder if we go overboard on that when it comes to Sunday worship. Becky McDaniel muses that part of raising a child in the church tends to include clothing them in their "Sunday best" and training them to sit still and quiet in a pew—and to do so under penalty of death, so to speak. But many children by their nature tend not to be polished and pristine dressers. At their most natural, they tend to be disheveled, noisy, and squirmy. If a child's only experience of church worship is as a training ground for bodily self-control, is it any wonder they become young adults who are turned off by church and do not think of their bodies as divine dwelling places? If our actions unwittingly teach children that God only likes their bodies if they are clean, tidy, restrained, and well-dressed according to adult standards, is it any wonder they become young adults who distrust that God wants good things for them?

Jonathan Thomas maintains that one should not downplay the power of the space itself to teach theologically. Like other clergy who have invited yoga into their worship spaces, he notes how healing it is for people who have felt wounded by a religious institution to bring their bodies (which in some cases have been shamed) to practice yoga in the worship space of a Christian church.

Caroline Kramer used meditation and art to shift the focus of spirituality away from the conventional "neck up–only" approach and into the entire body. Yoga was a natural next step after that. Diana Gustafson used the doctrine of the Incarnation to help her parishioners understand why yoga was being offered in the church worship space. Far from being just another new age fad, she taught that yoga has a place in Christian worship, since the God we worship chose to dwell in our human flesh, in the physical body of Jesus. This lays the foundation for the physicality of Christianity.

She notes that since the Enlightenment we have largely lost the theological primacy of the divine spirit within the physical body. Yoga can help reclaim this, and the asanas can be seen as spiritual exercises one does with the physical body. Our bodies are thus part of our spiritual selves. Diana cites the physicality of the worship of the Desert Fathers and Mothers, part of our spiritual heritage we are just beginning to reclaim. The movement of the human body is its own kind of prayer.

8. Leaders who welcome yoga into their churches are committed to respectfully maintaining the separate integrity of yogic philosophy and Christian theology–and yet are willing to take some risks, weaving together elements of Christian worship and prayer with yogic practice.

Becky McDaniel is a cradle Episcopalian who is comfortable challenging Episcopal orthodoxy—not for the sake of being ornery, she explains, but for the sake of reaching the lost and for the sake of reconciling people to God, each other, and themselves.

When Becky taught yoga at the seminary she attended, she used recordings of monastic chants, especially the hauntingly lyrical music of the twelfth-century Christian mystic Hildegard of Bingen, which can readily be found online. Becky didn't use the mantra *Om*, did engage a little theology and some mystical Christian poetry, and didn't tend to cite scripture. If she offered a didactic, it was short so that ample room could be left for silence. She notes we are much better at speaking to God than we are to listening. Reflecting on her own teaching style over the years, she acknowledges that in her first years she was much more loquacious than now.

At St. Catherine's Episcopal School, students love the opportunity for quiet that her yoga classes provide. The chapel is mostly dark, lit by candles. Taizé music might be playing. A screen might project a peaceful image from the natural world. She marks the beginning and end of the class with a Tibetan singing bowl. Other than these things, there is mostly silence.

Caroline Kramer experimented and yet had clear boundaries. She felt that if yoga was to be taught in the church as an act of worship, the theological language used would be Christian. Hindu gods would not be promoted or worshiped as some viable alternative to the Christian God. It was important to Caroline to hold her parish's story and character foremost in mind and not promote anything that felt out of accord with that.

Each class might have a broad theme and then a small bit of Christian content (scripture or poetry) in support of that theme. Caroline explored combining yoga and the Daily Office of Compline, but it didn't work as smoothly as she wished. She may try that again, breaking the Compline service apart and interspersing the component pieces with a vinyasa flow. She also teaches other yoga classes with Christian themes on the church campus.

Michael Sniffen found a yoga teacher who was a Roman Catholic. She asked him, "Do you want me to modify [Christianize] my language when teaching?" Michael told her no, asking her to be authentic to herself and to the tradition of yoga. He did not feel a need to "protect" Christianity by screening out insights from other philosophical or faith traditions.

At Grace Cathedral, yoga classes incorporate "universally resonant themes . . . of social justice and spiritual growth."[7] Jude Harmon will speak on a theological theme, drawing in both Christian theology and yogic philosophy, as we do at St. John's. A key difference is that his one teaching is less than five minutes, while ours have been longer. Harmon's teaching may be followed by a teaching of similar length from the yoga teacher. Aside from that, the class is all about movement, meditation, pranayama, and silence.

Because Cathedral Yoga at St. Mark's prioritizes contemplation over verbal didactic, they don't typically include readings or teachings as part of the class format. That said, they also leave much to the discretion of the teacher, wanting the teacher to do what feels authentic for them. A teacher might draw on a theme from a Sunday sermon but would be less likely to read scripture supporting that theme. One Cathedral Yoga teacher included a fair bit of social justice verbal teaching in

---

7. Andrea Rice, "San Francisco's Grace Cathedral Fosters Inclusivity and Healing Through Yoga," *Yoga Journal*, September 27, 2020, *https://www.yogajournal.com/lifestyle/san-franciscos-grace-cathedral-fosters-inclusivity-and-healing-through-yoga/*.

their class. It drew those looking for that kind of experience. Overall, however, organizers want to avoid coming off as preachy and note that such a stance can be polarizing, which would be at odds with their greater mission of hospitable inclusivity. Irene Beausoliel observes that Eastern yoga tends to emphasize philosophical teaching, while Western yoga leans more toward doing, or asanas. This is a generalization, of course, but Cathedral Yoga organizers are careful to teach to the audience that is before them, and that audience is Western influenced.

Diana Gustafson has been teaching yoga prayer services for about five years, drawing on the Daily Office of Evening Prayer. She uses the Book of Common Prayer and the New Zealand Prayer Book. It is an unmistakably Christian service but welcomes anyone. She sees her classes including as much prayer as they do yoga flows. A typical class composition might be twenty minutes of yoga, ten minutes of guided meditation, and some *Lectio Divina* (perhaps using a poem), not necessarily in this order.

9. Leaders who welcome yoga into their churches are not discouraged by resistance or obstacles.

Each of the individuals I talked with undertook some measure of preemptive education or formation with their congregations, either prior to launching a yoga ministry or concurrent with it. In some cases, this was part of a broader catechetical approach to leadership. Such an approach means the church is committed to forming disciples and uses liturgy, teaching, pastoral care, fellowship, ministries of serving and justice—everything—to create what's been called a *catechumenal metabolism*. Healthy churches have such a metabolism, recalling that in the early church, Christians were made, not born. Leaders of healthy churches seek to lead according to that way of understanding.[8]

The clergy bringing yoga into their worship spaces also tend to view operational glitches not as roadblocks but as obstacles they need to step over or around—or even signals from the Spirit to proceed ahead in a slightly different way.

When Michael Sniffen first visited the Cathedral of the Incarnation, he found a 500-seat, nineteenth-century French Gothic worship space with seventy-foot high ceilings. The floor space was pew-bound, with pews all the way up to the chancel. Imagining the possibilities for the space, he removed the first ten rows of pews. *Gasp.* Haven't ecclesial wars been waged over such things?

8. The Rev. Dr. Patricia Lyons, keynote address, October 4, 2019, Episcopal Diocese of Colorado annual convention.

Michael didn't take this action impulsively. He brought his PhD in ritual theory and liturgical studies to bear. He unearthed and studied the cathedral's original architectural drawings and realized it had been designed in the style of European cathedrals—to be a worship space without pews. His academic credentials and careful research helped cathedral members release the idea that the pews were part of some original and divinely ordained design.

Although there was not widespread pushback, there were plenty of questions. People wanted to know how, as a new dean, yoga fit into his overall vision for the cathedral. Michael chose to teach nondefensively around it, saying that all things in the worship space each in their own way supported some aspect of the Incarnation. In other words, God was equally glorified by high church services and by Community Food Share, both of which happened in the space.

In conversation with a handful of cathedral members, he asked them, "Could you imagine yourself in this space, looking up at the ceiling far above, and practicing yoga?" The responses ranged from moderate interest to seeing no connection between the soaring airspace of the cathedral and the soaring possibility of divine union offered by yoga. He did not permit this mixed initial response to halt his plans, but several months into the new yoga ministry he did make a point of checking in; he went back and revisited the topic with the cathedral yogis. All had come to embrace the sacred possibilities of doing yoga in the worship space.

One common misconception is that a cathedral, by virtue of its grandeur, is financially well endowed, for ever and ever, amen. The same misconception is often held regarding large downtown churches of beautiful architecture. Seldom do people stop to consider the fantastic operating costs of these massive structures. At Grace Cathedral, Jude Harmon was obliged to confront a potential downside of the cathedral's thriving yoga ministry: imagine an extra 800 people using the restrooms every week and the impact that has on water, wastewater, utility, janitorial, and supply costs. How does a cathedral or a parish church lower the barriers to the community's participation in a ministry—offering it at no-cost or for a freewill donation—and yet still offset the impacts those ministry participants have on the calendar, life, and budget of the church?

It sounds like a cold analysis to undertake, but unless it is conducted, there is real potential for misunderstandings. Before a yoga in the worship space ministry ever begins, church leaders and yoga teachers need to be in philosophical agreement about what a yoga ministry is trying to accomplish and what concessions each party—yoga teacher and church leader—is willing to make to ensure the ministry's success. The more well-known a yoga teacher is in the community, the more people they will attract, and inevitably the church may have to cede control over every detail of the ministry. This means that establishing a shared vision and good lines of communication are critical long before the first mat is ever unrolled.

It's tempting to let ministries arise organically. After all, isn't that how the Spirit works? The answer is yes—but a qualified yes. God gave us leaders the brains and gifts of discernment to see beyond the immediate: to vision, strategize, and imagine the problems we might need to confront. As appealing as it is to let a ministry grow completely on its own, it is vital for church leaders to supply the framework within which it can grow well.

That became part of Jude's job when he arrived at Grace—to build a framework for yoga. That meant things like working with the fire marshal to assure lanes of egress remained open, creating intake forms for yogis, designing a system for donations, recruiting and training volunteers to help, deciding who would manage advertising, and visioning how yoga should fit in with the cathedral's other ministries. It takes three hours every week just to set up the worship space for yoga, so building a network of helpers was essential.

At St. Mark's their long-running and much-loved Choral Compline service, in which attendees are free to lie down on the pews or the floor, cleared the way for creative use of the worship space. But Cathedral Yoga was not immune to criticism. When the ministry began, a handful of people were uneasy about the close proximity of yogis to the altar. Several times, community members wandered in to pray, found Cathedral Yoga in progress, and were unhappy not to have the space to themselves. Cathedral Yoga's organizers discovered that even non-church members have opinions about what should and shouldn't take place in a worship space. The yoga teachers handled these issues promptly, directly, kindly, and respectfully as they arose.

In 2019 the cathedral replaced many of its pews with chairs, which would afford much greater use of the nave floor space. The pandemic hit before Cathedral Yoga could really take advantage of this new flexibility of space. It's one of the things organizers look forward to when the yoga ministry resumes.

The city of Seattle is part of a metropolitan area with a population approaching four million. In addition to the typical noise of urban life, the cathedral sits uphill from the I-5 expressway, is on a flight path for the SEA-TAC airport, and picks up noise from float planes taking off from nearby Lake Union. Cathedral Yoga organizers engage soft music to cover or offset noise distractions. What some might see as an obstacle to contemplative practice they see instead as an opportunity to enhance the practice with music.

When Caroline Kramer launched a yoga ministry at her church, she was mindful of the ministry "turf" that existed in the church before she came. She took care to honor this and make clear to folks that although meditation, for example, might be part of a yoga workshop, she was not seeking to compete with or supplant existing meditation ministries. People tend to be protective of the ministries they build or lead. It's important to respect their work by explaining ahead of time how yoga fits in to what is already going on in the parish.

Caroline had to work out a payment arrangement with the yoga teacher. There's no one right answer to whether or how to charge for a Yoga in the Church class and whether or how to compensate a teacher. Here are some considerations:

- Is the teacher a parishioner, and does she or he consider teaching part of their Christian ministry? Or is she or he a community member who needs to be paid to help make a living?
- Do church leaders feel strongly that Yoga in the Church should be free? If so, are they willing to underwrite the cost of paying a teacher?
- Is a teacher willing to gamble that she or he will be compensated fairly and adequately if the church establishes a pay-what-you-can rule? Is the church willing to underwrite the difference if donations fall short of the expected fee?
- If the church cannot underwrite a teacher with cash, might they do so by offering that teacher a rent-free classroom or parish hall to teach another "regular" yoga class during the week?

Whatever is decided, it's not a bad idea to let the parish know how the teacher is being paid and why. If the vision is to offer a free or pay-what-you-can class, leaders need to be able to articulate and defend that vision to the parish. Being transparent about this upfront can avoid murmuring about fairness down the road. Be aware that precedents are easily set and, once rooted, tend to live in parish memory forever.

10. Leaders who welcome yoga into their churches tend to place a value on the sanctity of silence and contemplation.

At St. John's, contemplation is in the DNA of the congregation. It was there before I arrived and will probably be there long after I am gone. I didn't create it; I was simply smart enough to spot it and build on it. St. John's supports several Centering Prayer groups, a labyrinth, a contemplative Evensong, a service of choral Compline, an Intentional Community (a group of parishioners who developed and follow a rule of life), and a silent Maundy Thursday–Good Friday all-night watch.

Early on in my liturgical presidership, I began observing—*really* observing—the silences suggested by the rubrics in the Book of Common Prayer service of Holy Eucharist: after the Lessons, before the Confession of Sin, and at the Breaking of the Bread. At St. John's, we introduce the Confession by saying, "Let us confess our sins against God and our neighbor, *first taking a few moments to reflect in silence*." We even maintained this invitation to Confession when the pandemic obliged us to take worship online. When I first introduced silence into our liturgy I expected some objection, but no one squawked. On Sundays, no one fidgets or coughs loudly to signal their disapproval. I knew I was in the company of a congregation that naturally values the vital role of silence in worship. It was thus not a huge leap for this congregation to understand the sanctity that attends the silent practices of yoga. They already had a built-in respect for them. This is a useful study to undertake before bringing yoga into your church. How much silence in worship are you already observing?

I appreciate the creative ways clergy are inspired to draw on yoga as they lead Sunday worship. Ann Gillespie has taught an instructed Holy Eucharist in which she uses a heart-opening yoga asana during the "Lift up your hearts" of the *Sursum Corda*. Diana Gustafson wrote her seminary honors thesis on the contrast between the *Om* of yogic philosophy and the Great AMEN in the Episcopal eucharistic liturgy. What if, she muses, we taught people that the Great AMEN is the sound of the universe, like *Om*? I was taught that this amen is the only text in the entire prayer book in all capital letters. It is printed thus to underscore that it is a hearty and joyous affirmation to the eucharistic act. Sadly, we tend to say it rather tentatively, because somewhere in our distant pasts someone told us it wasn't seemly to be exuberant in church.

Diana said that people write to her to tell her that her yoga classes have opened their spiritual lives. She wonders aloud, "What if every church worship service gave people that same experience of opening their hearts; of generosity in action; of welcome?" She explains the act of palming (rubbing the palms together vigorously) and then placing the palms over the eyes (part of what some yoga teachers know as *Kapal randhra dhauti*, or skull-cleanser practice). When the palms are removed, yogis are invited to turn to their neighbors, greet them, and thank them for being part of the day's practice. What might it be like to incorporate this into the practice of Passing the Peace?

11. Leaders who welcome yoga into their churches recognize the potential of yoga to help shape the congregation's identity and sense of community.

Through their online presence, many churches proclaim that they are welcoming and inclusive. But if and how they live that out in their common life is sometimes less clear. When I visit a church's website, I look less at what they say about themselves and more at what they do. Does support for the poor and marginalized consist of financial donations, or do they get involved in serving with their hands and bodies? Do their ministries tend to favor fellowship and formation or hands-on work in poor and marginalized communities? Are they active in social justice? Sometimes such ministries can provide gentle doorways into the life of the church for those disinclined to enter through the red doors on a Sunday morning. When ministries like yoga are welcome and advertised, it tells the public (and reminds parishioners) that this church provides a home for a diversity of people and perspectives. As Paul said, the gospel is for both Jews and Gentiles—for those who believe and those who, God willing, will eventually come to do so.

At St. Mark's Cathedral, Greg Bloch observes that the mere presence of Cathedral Yoga in the worship space says something important about who St. Mark's is and that the very fact that Cathedral Yoga exists may make the cathedral more appealing to young people, even if they never attend. He dreams that the yoga ministry will grow ever more integrated into the cathedral's offerings and will attract more parishioners. He notes that the fact that the cathedral website lists Cathedral Yoga as one of their Sunday liturgical or worship opportunities says a great deal about how the cathedral defines *worship*. It may seem a mere detail of website architecture, but it is an important witness to the cathedral's expansive sacramental theology.

For Michael Sniffen, Mark Genszler, and Jonathan Thomas and Jenny Replogle, a ministry of yoga was part of the revitalization of the churches they served. Yoga was one part of the larger transformation of St. Luke and St. Matthew, from a congregation focused on survival to one focused on flourishing. Yoga likewise was part of the shift in identity at St. Paul's, from cathedral to parish and from ownership to belonging. Jonathan Thomas hopes the surrounding community can come to see St. Paul's as an entity that cares for and about people beyond its membership roster—a church that cares for the *whole* person and wants to help provide for their rest and healing. He hopes the community can find sanctuary at St. Paul's in the broadest sense of the term.

Church of the Holy Comforter worked for many years to plan and build a large ministry center on the church campus. It became the Center for Wellness and Spirituality and is an important statement about the parish's identity. Ann Gillespie had just brought yoga to the center when the pandemic hit. Other healing and wellness practices there include Reiki, pastoral counseling, and spiritual direction. Some of this ministry continued online during the months of church closure. When the pandemic abates, one aim will be to reach people who might not otherwise set foot in a church. Again, a gentle doorway.

Diana Gustafson once took a studio class that was fairly crowded. Someone came in quite late. The teacher stopped and asked the class to move their mats and make space for the latecomer. The teacher said, "You don't know what this person had to do to get here today." It invited Diana to resist the natural human inclination to be judgmental and to assume the worst of the latecomer—that they were a thoughtless person. It led her to ponder how she and her congregation might cultivate this same attitude of compassionate welcome on Sunday morning.

Smaller yoga classes seem to form their own communities. In larger yoga gatherings, building a sense of community may require a little structure and encouragement. At Grace Cathedral, the leadership wondered how it might help foster a sense of community and connectedness among the 800 yoga attendees. They encouraged and resourced the formation of small groups to provide a place for attendees to gather after class and discuss more deeply the theme or teaching that had been presented. Supporting the formation of these groups was an inspired idea. They drew fewer than fifty people and didn't seem to catch on in a big way, perhaps because (by virtue of being scheduled immediately following class) they cut into the dinner hour. Sometimes even inspired ideas need tweaking and restarts before they can take root.

Members of the cathedral's congregation council came to yoga to experience the class and to better understand the ministry. They understood the value of building a sense of community among this yoga congregation. A ministry budget was established, and three annual fellowship gatherings were offered to the yoga attendees. One event is Yoga for Change, which raises money for tuition assistance, meals, and learning materials for a San Francisco preschool. Yoga for Change has been taking place for eight years and engages the yoga congregation in a ministry of charitable giving. It also offers them a common purpose and helps build a sense of identity.

At St. Mark's Irene Beausoliel appreciates that Cathedral Yoga builds community in the moment and asks no long-term commitment of its members. While this is quite different from building a sense of community in a church congregation—where we pray for and promote a person's long-term commitment—it is a no less valid expression of shared values and behaviors. Might the church come to regard both temporary in-the-moment communities (those who show up for a yoga class) *and* cradle-to-grave communities (those lifelong parishioners who comprise a cherished subset of the church membership roster) as equally marvelous expressions of the work of the Spirit in the Church?

12. Leaders who have welcomed yoga into their churches reflect that it has been a holy process.

We're all servants who do various things to build up the church, said Paul to the Christians at Corinth (1 Cor. 3:6). I plant, Apollos waters, but it is God who gives the growth. Paul doesn't say it, but I'll bet you, he, and Apollos watched eagerly for God to do the divine work. I bet they grabbed each other's forearms and jumped up and down with glee when they saw that first green shoot. And I bet as the plant (the infant church) grew up, Paul and Apollos continually gasped with wonder as they witnessed the Spirit midwifing something new. That's the way I see these inspirational yogi priests and lay leaders who plant and water. They hold a sense of wonder at what God is doing in their churches. They cultivate the language to name it. They regard glimpsing the work of the Spirit in this yoga ministry as a privilege and gift.

Church leaders make hundreds of operational decisions every week: what color to repaint the nursery, whether to print worship bulletins on recycled paper, what topic this year's Lenten formation series should highlight, which scripture texts to preach on, and who might best fill an empty seat on vestry. Make no mistake: God is in all these discernings, and some have theological import. But in and of themselves they are more operational than theological. Bringing yoga into the worship space is quite different. It is a theological decision with operational implications. Because of that, it makes sense to pray about it with a greater depth of intention and attentiveness. Those attitudes shouldn't fall away once the yoga ministry has been launched. Pay attention, and you will be gifted and privileged to watch the Spirit at work before your eyes.

Mark Genszler can point to the genesis of his church's yoga ministry. It was in part his own desire together with his trust in a loving God that sparked the idea. When he went inward in prayer to search his heart, what he found was that what fed him was what God wanted for his parish. God does God's work in the world using whatever happens to interest or light us up. What a profound statement that is about the kind graciousness of God.

As Yoga at Grace grew to draw hundreds of attendees every week, Jude Harmon stood outside Grace Cathedral and watched people arrive. He said the sight of people streaming up the steps to the cathedral on a Tuesday night brought to mind the homecoming described in Isaiah 60:3–4: "Nations shall come to your light, and kings to the brightness of your dawn. Lift up your eyes and look around; they all gather together, they come to you." He had a clear sense he was witnessing something holy—God at work in the world before his eyes. Isaiah's description of homecoming, over 2,500 years old, was being translated freshly before him. Through yoga, Grace Cathedral drew the community to itself, and Yoga at Grace became a pilgrimage destination for people from as far away as Europe.

Becky McDaniel witnessed the power of God working through yoga to heal people and communities. Before discerning for the priesthood, she taught yoga, specializing in yoga for survivors of trauma, children with autism and anxiety disorders, the elderly, and teens. From there she began serving as a hospice volunteer and first heard a call to ordained ministry. She became interested and involved in Wisdom Schools, rooted in the wisdom tradition of Christianity. When she eventually went to seminary, Becky could see how God had been present in her vocational journey and in her yoga teaching, and was using one to inform the other.

As the daughter of an Episcopal priest, Ann Gillespie considered the priesthood well down on the list of possible life vocations. But yoga turned out to be a big part of her becoming a priest. It thawed her resistance to institutional religion and enabled her to develop a spirituality in her body. It was this that finally made room for her to hear and take seriously God's call to ordained ministry.

Diana Gustafson and Jonathan Thomas found that their yoga ministries enriched their own understandings of the theology of the Incarnation. Michael Sniffen invited his congregation to think of worshiping "beyond words" and encouraged them to "let their bodies *be* the prayer." He realized that we share in divinity not because we might be generous or loving or compassionate or disciplined or afire for social justice, but simply by virtue of being incarnate. This is perhaps one of the greatest gifts of the Christian faith: we share in divinity simply by virtue of being incarnate. Never forget that when the clouds broke apart, the light streamed through, the Spirit descended like a dove, and the voice of God said, "Oh, dear one of my own, how I love you! How well you please me!" Jesus had not yet performed miracles or healings. He had not taught, led, or inspired. All he did was stand up. To do that in yoga is called *tadasana*, or mountain pose. It is a way of saying with your body, "I am." I *am*. For God, that brings great joy and is more than enough.

EPILOGUE

> What we call the beginning is often the end
> And to make an end is to make a beginning.
> The end is where we start from . . .
> With the drawing of this Love
> And the voice of this Calling
> We shall not cease from exploration
> And the end of all our exploring
> Will be to arrive where we started
> And know the place for the first time.[1]
>
> –*T. S. Eliot*

A Yoga Prayer for the Church

When our anxious eyes see only the death of what we love,
Let our hearts see deeper and perceive the resurrection you embed in each dying.
For you told us, "Behold, I am doing a new thing!"
May the seeds we plant serve your work, O Lord.
Let us find joy in the labor of planting and release the expectation of harvest.

Remind us of your immanence, that you are as close as our breath.
Let our curiosity out-measure our fear
So we might stop clinging to what was and journey toward what shall be.
May we find you waiting there for us, delighted that we have come.
Draw us out of the comfortable nests of our intellect
and into the wilderness of our bodies.
Let those bodies be our prayer to you—sufficient, pleasing, and whole.

If you are the roaring ocean, the flowing river, the tranquil pond at dawn,
Then we are drops of You within you.
Bring us often to the still place and grant us self-compassion.
Let us claim our birthright as mystics.
Guide our feet to the high-arched and humble bridge

1. Four Quartets, T.S. Eliot, epigram drawn from "Little Gidding," IV.V, *http://www.davidgorman.com/4quartets/*.

Where we might meet the other and learn from him
So that we may know you better.

You break boundaries,
and yet we erect fences
Around our faith traditions to protect their purity,
which we call "orthodoxy"—an elegant name.
Let us instead allow you to protect your own Church,
And make us way-finders—
Celestial navigators in small boats
Following your great Spirit.

Let our bodies serve as altars where we worship you.
When you tell us in the Eucharist that you gave your body for us
Let us receive that gift saying,
"And here is *my* body, dear Lord, given for *you*."
Let there be a reciprocity of grace.

You whose thoughts are not ours,
You whose ways are higher than our own:
Remind us always that our bodies
(Imperfect, frail, flawed,
Not as we might wish them to be,
Nor as the world tells us they ought to be)
Are your manger and your home.
Remind us you see fit for them to hold Paradise.

Give us the courage to wade into the confluence
And the strength to stand in its turbulence.
With you, let us make holy the ground
Let us Christify the earth and all that is therein.

Give us the eyes to see the way you open before us.
When obstacles arise, fill our lips with your words
That we might teach around them.
Use us, we humbly pray, to help heal the wounds
Our very Church has inflicted.
Bless us in the work of restoration.
And in all things may we and the whole world
Find and dwell in union with you. *Amen.*

—*The Rev. Susan W. Springer*